Endorsements for

"This timely book is packed with [...] on how we can best advocate [...] f a loved one. Written in Reina's warm, engaging and supportive voice, it is peppered throughout with relevant and often humorous personal anecdotes. I have no doubt that following Reina's counsel will lead you to improved health outcomes. There's plenty of great advice for health care professionals as well, from a very experienced and articulate patient."

—*J. Noe, PharmD BCOP, Co-owner PDstat*

"Reina's book really nicely summarizes her lessons learned from years of accumulated experience as both a patient and a healthcare professional. This is a helpful read for anyone with a complex, chronic illness that requires lots of contact with the medical community."

—*Sascha Tuchman, MD, Associate Professor and Director of the UNC Multiple Myeloma and Amyloidosis Program*

"I have known Reina as a friend for 45 years. She is knowledgeable, capable, and caring.

When my significant other was recently diagnosed with lung cancer, Reina was the first person I called. She was still weak from having her own chemo treatments but she drove some distance to give him (and me) reassurance, information, and most importantly—comfort.

Another plus—she has a great sense of humor!"

—*N. Allison*

"Just before my emergency surgical procedure I remembered Reina Weiner's advice to "trust your doctor, but not that much." I questioned my doctor regarding a pre-op procedure. He made a change and all went well. Thanks, Reina, for helping me be "my own, best healthcare advocate."

—*E. Puening*

"Reina is one of the strongest, most inspirational people I know."

—*L. Grubman*

"This book reads like you are listening to a good friend who is giving you wise and loving advice. The author encourages you to advocate for yourself and gives you great suggestions on how to become an active participant in your own healthcare. With all it's serious points, it's got some humor in it as well. The smart advice at the end of each chapter summarizes the salient points that are easy to remember."

—*P. L. Joyce*

"In *Trust Your Doctor, But Not That Much!*, Reina Weiner shares with us the benefit of her experiences as a healthcare consumer and as one who has worked in the industry. The take home, as Reina reiterates throughout her text is, that we should all advocate for ourselves when our health and well-being are at stake. Our very lives can be at risk. We can't assume or trust that it will always be done for us. Reina provides us with the tools and incentive to advocate for ourselves. I recommend that not only healthcare consumers read the book, but also healthcare providers as it provides opportunity for reflection with regard to how we are perceived by our patients. Pick up a copy and read it today, "why wait?"

—*Kathy Carroll, N.P.*
fellow clinical trials participant

"Remarkably candid and helpful advice on how to collaborate with your doctor! A perfect gift for someone with any new diagnosis."

—*W. Victoria Morehouse, M.D.*
(Board Certified in Pediatrics and Internal Medicine)

"Reina has been my patient and friend for more than 7 years. The first time we met she asked me what we could offer and why she should stay with our program. I could tell she had done her homework. She also told me that she needed my help as a specialist, to give recommendations and to provide care, treatment and follow-up. Just like life in general, due to Reina's disease, we have gone through both hard and easier times together. In my eyes, Reina was born with a positive way of looking at life with lots of energy that keeps her going. Her family is always there for her. The energy, positive thinking, and family support are all key ingredients in life—particularly when diagnosed with cancer. This amazing book provides a unique perspective—from the inside—of being diagnosed with cancer, going through therapy, with the attendant recommendations, care, treatment and follow-up. It is hands-on with valuable advice while still keeping a positive outlook on the future. Every person diagnosed with cancer and every doctor treating cancer patients should read this book!"

—*C. Ola Landgren, M.D.,*
Professor of Medicine
Chief, Myeloma Service
Department of Medicine
Memorial Sloan Kettering Cancer Center

Trust Your Doctor...
but Not That Much

To Marty,
A wonderful, healthcare
advocate.
Best,
Reina S. Weiner

Trust Your Doctor...
but Not That Much

Be Your Own Best Healthcare Advocate

REINA S. WEINER

This book is not intended as a substitute for the medical advice of a physician. The reader should regularly consult with a physician in matters relating to his/her health and particularly with respect to any symptoms that may require diagnosis or medical attention.

www.reinaweiner.com

ISBN: 978-578-43314-10

Publisher: Why Wait, LLC
Cover design: Christy Collins, Constellation Book Services

Printed in the United States of America

Contents

Preface

Why Have I Written This Book

It's funny how life moves you in different directions, but still along the same path. That's how it's been for me.

I've had a lifelong interest in medicine. First, I worked as a medical assistant/secretary in doctor's offices and hospitals in several states, then as a contract pharmaceutical representative and thereafter, as an oncology representative. As an oncology representative my role was to understand and effectively present clinical trials papers to doctors, nurse practitioners, oncology nurses and pharmacists. Part of those presentations involved a discussion of the most effective ways to manage side effects from chemotherapy. Years later when I became a national oncology trainer, I clearly recognized a well known truism—the more you teach, the more there is to learn. My teaching/learning experience was augmented for several years as an Adjunct Associate Professor for nursing students. Working for and with healthcare practitioners has given me both an understanding and an insider's view of the profession. The work is not easy and most often, not very glamorous.

In spite of the above experiences I've had, there are several questions that keep popping up in my head: Why don't people trust themselves enough at home, at work, as a parent, and as a patient to ask for what they need? Asking for what you need, why wait and trusting yourself—were all born in printed, e-book and spoken word format from those personal, recurring questions. Trusting yourself as a parent and learning to trust your kids became my first book, *Strong From the Start—Raising Confident and Resilient Kids.*

My work experience and personal journey led me to write what you're reading now—*Trust Your Doctor...but Not That Much—Be Your Own Best Healthcare Advocate.*

I come from both sides of medicine—initially facing the doctor across from his desk with a clinical paper in my hand—listening, talking, asking questions and later facing the doctor with my own notes and questions from the examining table as a patient in a clinical trial for cancer. Many years earlier I'd been there when both my parents had cancer surgeries simultaneously and for their aftercare as well. So, I get it.

My goal is never to undermine physicians. Their hope and intention have always been to cure and heal which is why they've trained so diligently in medical school and years thereafter. But with today's healthcare regulations, restrictions, and the "business of medicine," they are often rushed and overwhelmed.

My purpose in writing this book is to provide a roadmap so you, the patient, can get better healthcare. I also want to offer some support for what is an often confusing, circuitous, frustrating and difficult path. This book is not only for people who have cancer and other life-threatening diseases, it's for everyone who's ever been a patient with any health problem (great or small) or who's been a caregiver or supporter—the one who takes his kids or accompanies her parents to the doctor. My goal is to create mutual respect between the healthcare professionals and patients and open the door to more welcome questions that lead to beneficial, receptive, and responsive conversations. Most of all, I hope to encourage you, the patient, to feel empowered so you can get the answers and the treatment that you need and want.

CHAPTER 1

How Do I Find a Doctor/ Healthcare Professional?

Have you recently moved? Your physician has retired or no longer participates in your insurance plan? Need a specialist for a new problem? Or, your present healthcare provider no longer meets your needs, be they physical or emotional? Well then, how do you find the right healthcare professional for you?

1. Many of us have been or will find ourselves in this predicament in the future. Whether or not you have great insurance or are on Medicare/Medicaid, there are competent doctors or nurse practitioners out there who provide quality care. Here are a few tips as you begin your search.

- Know any nurses? Nurses are often well-informed and can be a good source for a physician, nurse practitioner (NP) or physician assistant (PA) referral. Their recommendations are based on professional experience so you can count on them to assess the competence of a physician, an NP or a PA. They have the inside scoop about who's who, if you know what I mean. Individuals who work directly with doctors are ideal people to ask for a referral. Your friendly nurse will save you time and energy by quickly eliminating a doctor who would not be right for you and instead recommend a healthcare professional who you may find is a great fit. *My point: Ask the people who know best—those who work directly with physicians/NP's/PA's.*

- Don't know any nurses personally? Consider calling the local hospital and ask for the Director of Nurses. I have made this call in the past. More recently, I've spoken with the Scheduling Office at my local hospital. They will provide a list of local doctors who are taking new patients. The staff will also schedule an appointment for you with a doctor. Alternatively, you can look up a doctor online, research his or her background, where the doctor has trained and then make an appointment with the doctor you've chosen.

- One of the best internists I've ever been the patient of was in San Antonio, Texas; he was referred to me by a nurse working in a different physician's office.

I don't know how long it would have taken me to find him without her recommendation. If you happen to be a patient of another specialty practice, i.e., a gynecologist, orthopedist, dermatologist, physical therapy, etc., consider asking the nurse/PT whom he or she would recommend. Pharmacists are also a great resource for physician/nurse practitioners. My compounding pharmacist was happy to share the names of several healthcare professionals when I asked him for a referral. Sometimes you have to take the long way around the block to find a great physician, but it's so worth the effort.

◆ Don't be shy about checking with the local nursing society in your area. Check out www.Nurses. org. This organization lists state nurse's chapters around the country. Call or email the group so you can make direct contact with a nursing professional. Also search for nurse practitioners in your community; they're listed in ANCC.org and www.Nurses.org. These are credentialed medical professionals who can write prescriptions whom you can visit for your general healthcare. So can P.A.'s. Check out NCCPA.net. Often, both NP's and PA's have more time than many physicians. If you're not ready to have a nurse practitioner or a PA as your primary healthcare provider, ask one for a referral to an internist/family practice doctor.

◆ Most counties within the U.S. have local medical societies. Try putting MedicalSociety of (your county). org—MedicalSocietyyourcounty.org—into Google to locate the medical society nearest you. You may find it necessary to put in your region rather than your county to find a physician. It's best to spend a little time on Google to gather the names of physicians you might like to see. It's time well spent. Additionally, check www.nmanet.org to look for physicians in your region. Representatives at medical societies are generally happy to recommend a local doctor. Do try to be as specific as possible about your needs—whether you'd prefer a group or solo practice or a doctor in a certain location. Discuss whether you'd like a male or female or a practice catering to a particular age group. Your input with appropriate details can help someone direct you to the right healthcare professional. Give your priorities some thought before you contact any professional organization that provides referrals.

- Ask a friend who has had previous experience with a doctor/nurse practitioner whom he or she has used. This recommendation may not lead to the right healthcare practitioner for you, but it's a way to begin your search. Most recently, I've chosen to try a doctor (and I do mean "try" a doctor to see if we can work together), referred by a neighbor. I'll have a visit with him and decide whether he's the right one for me. Remember, you have choices whether you have a preferred provider network or not. Consider other doctors, if after several visits, there isn't good chemistry between you and the physician.

- If your doctor is retiring, she may already have a physician to recommend. Be sure to ask. Or, if your doctor is part of a group practice, there may be another doctor in that practice you can try.

- Know your diagnosis? Google it—www.google.com—and see if any specialists located in your community have written about your diagnosis. WebMD, Mayo Clinic or Healthgrades are good sites to explore.

We've moved recently and have been going through the "search." Several physician names were offered by my new neighbors. Additionally, I called an ophthalmologist I had been to for a referral. His office quickly called me back with three names. Two of those doctors were not accepting any new patients, but one was. I scheduled an appointment with one of the doctors in the practice for myself and another one for my husband. (That's the office policy.) As it turned out, my husband's physician was smart, warm and a great fit for him. My doctor was also very competent, but not someone whom I felt very comfortable with at first, but I chose to give her a second chance. That has turned out to be a wise decision. She's a smart, capable, thorough physician. We've gotten to know one another better and now have a comfortable, easy rapport. Do give a physician another opportunity to get to know you better and you her after your first visit. You can always choose another physician, thereafter, if you feel you two are not clicking.

Because I was initially not sure I would continue to be a patient of doctor number one my next move was to contact a large, local, internal medicine practice. I spoke at length with the appointment scheduler letting her know my needs and asked who she would recommend. I've found most people will help you if you're sincere about wanting their help. We've scheduled an appointment. Doctor number two listened to my concerns and wrote several prescriptions I requested yet never examined me. He didn't even put a stethoscope on my chest, which I consider to be the very basics of an exam. I had to cross him off my list.

Your sense of trust and comfort with your physician is a significant element of good medical care. If that emotional comfort is not there with a specific doctor, don't be reluctant to look elsewhere. It's your choice. There's no need to create a big, dramatic scene in your doctor's office, if you're not satisfied with his or her care. You should simply go about finding someone more acceptable. And, don't be intimidated by friends/acquaintances/family who tell you how difficult it is to find a local family doctor or internist because of insurance, Medicare, Obamacare, an aging population in your community, practice limitations or the weather! Don't listen. Keep searching. Good medical care is out there, no matter where you live, if you take a little time to seek it out. By the way, it only took me one afternoon to get the names of several physicians in my area.

Here's a little aside. Quite a few years ago my husband's company went bankrupt. Money was tight. My internist didn't take insurance. Her office policy was that patients paid her directly and then were reimbursed by the insurance company. This was before I "grew up" and went on Medicare/supplemental insurance, which doesn't allow you to pay for healthcare services and then be reimbursed. I was hoping to keep her as my physician rather than find a new physician, if that was possible. I asked if she would accept my temporary insurance payment until we would be in better financial shape to pay her directly. Her response, "I'd rather sell shoes at Nordstrom than take insurance!" Pretty radical, right! But, although Nordstrom is a cool store with great shoes, I don't know any physicians who would shelve their licenses to sell shoes. Nonetheless, it seemed my only option was to find another doctor who would take my current health insurance. Then, a surprise. She didn't charge me for the visit. She chose to wait until we could afford to pay her directly as we always had in past years. Wow—an excellent physician with a great heart. This medical professional had the right combination of traits. Why did I tell you this story? Because if you find yourself in similar circumstances, don't hesitate to explain your situation to the doctor you've chosen. We all get in some sort of a bind occasionally. You may be pleasantly surprised at the generosity and commitment of your physician. And, just maybe you don't need to begin that search for a doctor who will take your current insurance after all.

- ◆ Sorry for the digression, but thought you might find the above anecdote useful. Back to more "finding a doctor suggestions." Corporations have recently gotten involved in managing healthcare practices. Your doctor may now be part of a multi-specialty group practice within a corporate structure. These types of physician practices often have a range of annual membership fees, in addition to patient visit fees. It can be pricey. But, if that works for you, your primary care doctor will easily be able to refer you to a specialist should that be necessary. Remember, it's only a referral, though not an obligation, and simply a place to begin. You may also want to switch to another primary care doctor or nurse practitioner within the group. Several doctors = several choices. Is a multi-physician practice a plus or a minus for you? You decide.

• There's also concierge medicine. You pay an annual retainer to have quick and unlimited access to your doctor. It's very personalized care. Several thousand dollars a year guarantees he or she will call you back shortly, or email/text you regarding your healthcare concerns. There is a charge for each office visit as well. It's not for everyone, but for some it provides the access they desire and the quality healthcare they're seeking. That's not to say it's necessary to become a patient of a concierge medical practice to receive good health care. Good care is available in all types of medical practices throughout the country. It may take a little longer for a healthcare professional to return your calls or email you through a patient portal due to a greater number of patients being cared for, but he or she will get back to you. Duke Integrative Medicine in Durham, N.C., near where I've lived for a time, is a concierge practice that incorporates complementary and traditional medicine.

The tranquil setting and the architecture alone automatically improve how you feel before you even step into the doctor's office! Unfortunately, it was too costly for me, although I'm pretty sure I would have loved being a patient there. It's a great practice, but I ended up finding very good healthcare in a more traditional medical office.

◆ Consider asking a pharmacist at your local pharmacy which doctor he or she would choose. Pharmacists speak with doctors, doctor's offices and nurse practitioners all day long. They get a sense of which doctor has the most well-organized practice, how the doctor handles misunderstandings should they occur, and who is the most knowledgeable. They're an excellent source to query for a referral.

2. When you think you've found a doctor or nurse practitioner you'd like to work with, set up an appointment for an interview, assuming the practice is accepting new patients. Not all practices will allow you to interview the physician, nurse practitioner, or physician assistant, but if they do, it's a terrific way to learn the healthcare professional's philosophy and how he or she interacts with patients, i.e., who contacts you with test results, which insurance is accepted, how referral appointments are made, how prescription refills are handled, and how you contact the doctor directly. If the practice doesn't allow interviews—my new doctor doesn't— you can make an appointment for a simple blood pressure check just to meet her and to decide if she's going to be the one. You may need to pay for this visit, but it's well worth

the money. Although referrals and reviews from others are useful, your comfort and confidence level with a provider will guide your choice appropriately. Trust yourself.

SMART ADVICE

◆ Ask a nurse you or a friend knows. Nurses are a fantastic resource. Who better to ask for a physician referral than a healthcare professional who has worked with other healthcare professionals? Nurses have the inside scoop.

◆ Don't know a nurse? Call your local hospital and ask for scheduling or speak with the Director of Nursing. States may differ in this regard, but don't hesitate to check with your local hospital. In Florida, the RNs in the doctor's office told me they couldn't refer me to a family practice. But, the North Carolina hospital in my town offered several physician's names and would make an appointment for me, if I wanted one. Do ask. The worst they can say is they're not allowed to help you out. On to the next possibility.

◆ Check with a local medical society MedicalSociety yourcounty.org or www.nmanet.org—and ask for a referral within your community.

◆ Google internists in your community. See which names come up and check them out by calling the office and making an appointment to decide if this doctor or nurse practitioner is a good fit for you.

Online reviews can be helpful, but sitting down with a doctor directly will tell you what you *need* to know.

- Talk to your friends and ask them if they've found a healthcare professional they like. This has always been and still is a very productive way to find a doctor.

- Ask a pharmacist in your town for the name of a physician.

- Query your current doctor or nurse practitioner, if he or she is retiring. Who would he or she go to as a patient? Don't be shy.

- If your current doctor no longer takes your insurance, consider paying him out of pocket, that is, if you want to continue as his patient.

- Multi-specialty practices are ideal for referrals as are concierge practices. Ask, ask, ask.

- If you have a chronic health problem, be sure to check out specific non-profit organizations, i.e., American Cancer Society, Susan G. Komen Women Breast Cancer, National Psoriasis Association, etc., that relate directly to an illness you may have. Again, spending some time doing online research to find non-profits, foundations, charities, etc. is a good idea. You'll be pleasantly surprised at what comes up. If you don't have a computer, go to a local library.

Even if you don't have a library card, you can use a computer there. And, if you're not a computer whiz, ask your grandkids or a teen neighbor to help you get information online.

- Your church, temple, mosque or any other organization may have a resource center. Check it out.

CHAPTER 2
Preparing for an Office Visit

Before you set out to see your health care provider—whether it's your first visit or one of many with her—sit down with pad and paper, your smart phone, iPad, or computer and start writing a comprehensive list of your specific health concerns. The more you include, the more "clues" you'll be providing your doctor/detective. You should include:

1: Your symptoms: Describe in particular when and how they began and whether there was a precipitating event (i.e., accident or illness). Where is the pain or the problem? Can you point to it on your body? Be as specific as you can. Include every little detail you can recall. I just read about a patient whose illness was precipitated by bending down! Sounds like I'm making this up, right? Unfortunately, I'm not. If you pay attention to your body and what happens to you before, during and after a certain set of circumstances, providing this input to your physician can help your doctor make the right diagnosis.

2: What you've done to improve your symptoms: These may include prescription drugs as well as over the counter drugs, i.e., ibuprofen, wine/whiskey (no kidding!), chiropractic adjustments, massage, physical therapy, acupuncture, meditation, bedrest and sick time from work. If you can't remember the names of all of the drugs you've tried or can't spell or pronounce them, don't worry. If you've still got them, pop them into a little bag and bring them with you. Don't be embarrassed. I've seen plenty of patients sitting in waiting rooms with Ziploc bags full of prescription and non-prescription drugs. It's the most accurate way to let the doctor or nurse know exactly what you've been taking. If you haven't taken any medication or done anything to improve your symptoms, say that.

3: Duration of the above treatment (or none) to improve your symptoms. Try to remember how long you've been trying each treatment or taking each medication.

4: Have your symptoms improved simply with time? With treatment? Do they wax and wane? Have they gotten worse? How much worse? If you've been having pain, consider using the pain scale (1—the least pain; 10—unbearable pain) Additionally, it's useful to "paint a picture," tell your story in words, i.e., "when I bent over to pick up the laundry I couldn't get up" or "I had to hop into the woods off the trail to pee" or—you can fill in the blanks here!) You get the idea. Do your symptoms improve or worsen at any particular time of day? Tell your story clearly and completely.

5: Any other drugs—street drugs, herbal supplements, homeopathic medicines, etc.—you're using: Please do share those. They can play a part in the doctor's diagnosis and treatment of your ailment.

6: Any other recent illnesses or accidents? Even if they appear to have no relation to your current problem, briefly mention them anyway.

7: Changes in your diet/exercise regimen: Are you eating more or less? Different foods? Are you exercising more or less than in the past?

8: Big time stresses in your home/work life (either positive or negative experiences)—new marriage, divorce, school, death of a loved one, moving, broken heart, exciting new job, issues with your kids, layoff, bankruptcy? Do mention any and all of the above. As we all know, stresses aren't always good for us, but they're unavoidable and can be a contributing factor to your health problem.

9: Have you had this health problem before? Sit and think, think, think. Even if it's a tidbit of information and seems insignificant to you, write it down anyway. You never know if that one little scrap of data is just what the doctor ordered. This may help her help you.

I know. It's a lot to consider and takes plenty of time. You're worth it. I suggested creating a list to my friend, Amelia, who has been living with multiple sclerosis. She was "surprised at how effective and effortless it was." Her doctor was "relieved" Amelia had shown up with all the pertinent information.

After you've prepared your list, written it clearly and succinctly (be sure you and your doctor can read it), print a copy for yourself and one for her. Remove it from your printer and please remember to bring it with you! Put a reminder in your computer or write it on your palm but do remember to bring your list with you. It's better to have a printed copy than a list on your iPhone, iPad. Both you and your doctor can look at it simultaneously. A friend of mine wrote out one list that he held in his hand. His physician abruptly grabbed it out of his hand. I always print out two lists. If you've printed two lists, the issue of control can be avoided.

Here's what happened when I visited one of my doctors with my list:

Doctor: "Is there going to be a test?"

Me: "There could be a quiz, so do your best!"

All kidding aside, bringing two lists of your health issues (one for you and one for your healthcare provider) does set a tone for the visit. It demonstrates that you will be an active, informed participant in your healthcare. Plus, providing a clear picture of what's going on with your health can make a huge difference in the physician's detective work necessary to shed light on your problem. You will be saving both you and your doctor time so the doctor can focus on your problem and how best to help you.

Also, be sure to bring with you: X-rays (the actual film, not just the report), blood work results, pathology reports (some docs want the slides to look at themselves, not just the pathology reports), CT or MRI or any other scan or test results performed recently. Older reports are helpful as well as they serve as a baseline (a term often used in medicine to look at how you "were" previously) comparing now with before. Have a copy of all these results in hand to share with your doctor. *Always ask for a CD copy of x-rays/CT's, MRI's (before you leave the radiology office) rather than just the printed report.* Most offices will give you the disc (though occasionally you may have to pay a fee) and your physician will be glad to view the films herself. I will discuss more on keeping your own records in Chapter 16.

Make another list of your choices as they refer to your potential care: Are there treatments you would prefer to skip or others you would agree to? If you'd rather not have any further x-rays, steroids, say so. If you'd prefer to receive only holistic or complementary medications in addition to or instead of traditional medicine, let your healthcare professional know that too. Do you have any religious/ spiritual/cultural commitments that could influence your treatment choices? If so, mention them to your doctor.

If you're going to the doctor for a sprained ankle, you'll probably have a little more information than you need! Obviously, you'll want to adjust this list as it pertains to your present health issue, but don't omit any prior, related problems. It can be tricky. But, it's better to bring too much information than not enough. That being said, please try hard to stick to the salient points. Going on about your dog, sweet as he is, will only waste your time and that of the doctor.

How about a list of questions you might ask your physician? It's difficult to conceive of questions if you're not even sure what ailment you have. But, if you think it may be that old, recurring, sprained ankle, give some thought to several appropriate questions you'd like to ask. Obviously, it's better to ask your questions while you're still on the examining table or in the office looking at the doctor or nurse practitioner in the eye than by cell phone, email or fax. Pose your questions directly to your healthcare provider *before* he or she leaves the room or he/she puts his/her hand on the door knob and tries to escape!

SMART ADVICE

Make a list that includes:

- Symptoms
- Treatments you've tried
- Duration of treatments. Improvement or worsening of your condition
- Other illnesses or accidents—even though they may appear unrelated
- Diet/exercise changes
- Significant stresses (divorce, job loss, promotion, moving, loss of partner)
- Whether your problem is a recurrent one
- X-rays, CT or MRI scans (the actual films, not just the written report),

- Blood work results—
- Any religious choices that influence treatments
- Two copies of any questions you have; one is for you and one is for your doctor
- Stick to your healthcare issues (Not your dog, politics, TV, your kids, etc.).

CHAPTER 3

Scary Diagnosis:
After I Stop Shaking
What Do I Do Next?

What do you do when your doctor presents you with a scary diagnosis? I've had this experience myself so I get it. First you feel fear, anxiety and confusion. Then, when you begin breathing again, you hit the computer and start your research to learn more about what's happening within your body and again, try not to freak out. After a while, when you've amassed enough information (which may vary according to your individual needs) you can begin considering your options. Finally, you and your healthcare provider can jointly choose the path ahead.

Briefly, that's your path after a diagnosis but here's a more detailed look.

You've found a doctor with whom you're comfortable. You've written your list of concerns and questions and had your first visit. Then you get the call. She says, "We need to look into your symptoms a little further and schedule a test or two. Maybe some blood work, a CT scan, MRI or the dreaded biopsy." Uh, oh. You're already beginning to worry. She says it could be nothing, of course, but the problem needs to be checked out. Another uh, oh. Now you can't wait to get the tests done and hopefully, receive good news.

Then you get the phone call. "Please come into my office, Mary Lou, so we can talk about the results of your tests." Now you're really worried because you know when the doctor calls and asks you to come in, she's not calling to discuss the new fabric you chose for your dining room chairs. You're in panic mode. At the office, your doctor slowly, carefully explains that you have a serious, chronic ailment. Oh no! But, there is treatment for your problem. Did I even hear anything my doctor said after the word cancer? No. Not one word.

I remember very well how I felt. Many years ago, I got that very phone call followed by the emotionally paralyzing office visit. When you hear the word cancer, you're sure it's going to be the end of your life tomorrow. What could be more terrifying? I was grateful my husband was with me to hold my hand and more importantly, listen far more objectively.

If you get the "phone call," please remember to bring someone with you to the doctor's office. It can be a good friend, family member, spouse or anyone you feel will be a calm listener who will hear and remember what you probably won't. This individual will explain it all to you later. If you or your supportive friend can repeat back to the doctor **in your own words what he has said** *before* **you leave the office,** you'll both be on the same page. If your relative or friend can take notes, all the better. There's enough confusion with medical terms; the stress of bad news and then trying to remember it all can be extremely difficult. Therefore, if your friend or family member can write it down or record the doctor's words (with the doctor's permission, of course) those notes can be a remarkable memory aid. Don't be shy about asking your doctor either to repeat what she's saying or slow down a moment so your friend can get it all written or typed.

When you begin to exhale again and remove your shoulders from around your ears, that's when it's a good idea to learn more about your specific health problem. Education is your indispensable friend now, but beware, it can also be your worst, fear-inducing enemy.

Whatever you can learn about the specifics of your illness may be advantageous. Bear in mind, you can learn a lot, but you won't have anywhere near as much knowledge or expertise as your physician. Still, having a solid understanding of your illness and all treatment options will go a long way toward ensuring you'll receive excellent care. As long as you are not in an emergency situation, taking the time to learn about your illness is essential. I like to listen to webinars by physicians who discuss the newest treatments and research regarding my illness. Staying up to date and being well informed allows you to become a more confident, active participant in your healthcare choices.

A word of caution here—one that was shared with me by a smart, young doctor when I got the lousy news about a blood disorder—try to stay away from the overly dramatic, worst-cases scenarios you will likely come across on the web. They only serve to scare the daylights out of you which isn't what you need at this point. Besides, every person is unique and so is his or her illness. Your health trajectory can be far different, less complicated and potentially more responsive to treatment than the patient you're reading about. It's certainly a worthwhile goal for anyone who gets the "bad news" to become more knowledgeable about their new health challenge, but getting paranoid doesn't help you heal and empower you as a patient. It's best not to focus on overall survival statistics or complications. That's way too depressing and is not necessarily your healthcare journey.

If your diagnosis is cancer, you want it treated and hopefully cured right this very minute. Your brain is screaming, "get this cancer out of me." Who wouldn't feel that way under the circumstances? But, again, unless your physician says you must be treated immediately, you have at least a few days, a week or more to stare at your computer, breathe, meditate, have a glass of wine, eat a pint of ice cream, take a walk, talk with a friend, calm down and read everything you can about the clinical trials data, treatments and more that pertain to your condition. I've been there and I know exactly how hard it is but, please remember, the more you know, the more likely you'll be able to engage your doctor in insightful conversations about your illness, the possible treatment choices and your personal preferences. Becoming your own best healthcare advocate and participating in your care is best achieved when you've become more knowledgeable about your health. Besides learning that you have choices, you'll be taking an active role in returning your body to optimum health.

As I've said, knowledge is your best friend when dealing with a serious disease. So, you hit the Internet. Again, if you need to get help doing online research, don't be afraid to ask anyone. Really, whether you find a younger, computer savvy person or an older one, don't hesitate to ask for help. Don't be shy! In order to be an effective advocate for your health, you will want to educate yourself as thoroughly and as completely as possible. Asking someone who is agile on the computer is just plain smart!

Where to start your search? Google your illness. Click on well known, academic institutions—Mayo Clinic, Johns Hopkins, NIH (National Institute of Health), or WebMD, etc., all of which have well written, understandable explanations of your health problem. Often, you will see websites providing a great deal of useful information and guidance free, i.e., The American Cancer Society, American Diabetes Association, Arthritis Foundation, etc. Within those major categories you'll find sub-topic organizations for diagnoses pertinent to you, possibly your type of cancer, type 2 diabetes, rheumatoid or osteoarthritis. These are just a few examples. For people like me who have blood cancer, I've accessed the International Myeloma Foundation and The Multiple Myeloma Research Foundation. They've been generous with both their time and expertise. In addition, the emotional support they share is invaluable. **Most chronic illnesses have support organizations/non-profits. Do check them out online.** They can direct you to financial and emotional support as well as much more information about your particular disorder. *The more you know, the more empowered you'll be.* When you learn you're not the only one with a health challenge it can be very reassuring. It doesn't take away your health problem, but it does make you feel less alone. Having more current, detailed knowledge about my health issues helps me feel empowered. And that sense of empowerment encourages me to take an even more active role in the future directions we (my doctor and I) will choose.

Empowered patients are smart patients. You may have a health problem, but you are not powerless.

- Bring a friend or family member—a good listener—with you when your doctor will be explaining test results.

- Have your "good listener" take notes or record (with the physician's permission) what he or she is saying.

- Repeat back to the doctor what he or she said *before* leaving the office.

- Begin your research when you can exhale again! Learn everything you can about your illness. Not great on the computer? Get someone to help you, if necessary.

- Stay away from "worst case" scenarios on the Internet.

- Mayo/Hopkins/NIH/WebMD as well as disease specific non-profits are all reliable sources of information.

CHAPTER 4

Choosing a Doctor/Hospital after Your Diagnosis

With all your research, you know quite a bit more about your condition than you did before. Now, it's time to create your most comprehensive list of questions so you can locate the physicians who only treat patients with your diagnosis. Although there are many smart doctors, if you have a serious illness, it's wise to seek out the ones who only take care of people like you.

If surgery has been suggested as part of your treatment plan, here's *the* question you must ask of the surgeon: **"How many of these surgical procedures do you perform in a year?"** ASK THE QUESTION LONG BEFORE THE ANESTHESIA, please! I know those words may get stuck in your throat, but take one of those long, slow, meditation-like breaths and ask it. *This question is not a maybe,* *it's a must.* Without a doubt this is a potential "save your life" question. At the very least, it's a question that will ease much of your pre-treatment stress because you will know you're in the right hands. Although there's actually no *perfect* in medicine, the best doctors for you are the ones who treat your illness day in and day out. Generally speaking, because they limit their practice to a specific patient population, they know more about your condition than other physicians who aren't specialists. They've got the latest knowledge about your illness, challenges, the newest treatments and what to expect from those treatments—the positives and the negatives. They've heard just about everything related to your illness and know what to do especially if something unusual arises. As a rule, healthcare providers are bombarded with a daily deluge of new drugs, treatments, diagnoses, etc. which makes it nearly impossible for them to keep up. Picking a doctor who has performed your surgical procedure over and over again, and/or one who is very familiar with your illness and drug regimen is simply the smartest choice you can make. I can't emphasize this option enough.

Let's look at Mr. B's story. He had been coughing frequently all last year. Finally, he visited a local surgeon and was scheduled for surgery to remove an esophageal mass—the assumed cause of his cough. He never asked how many times the doctor had performed this procedure. (The answer to that question may have you putting your coat on and politely leaving the doctor's office.) Sadly, Mr. B's surgery did not go well. After his first surgery, Mr. B. chose to ask his doctor how many of these surgical procedures he performed each year? Dr. Smith's response: "One or two a year." Uh oh.

This one question will provide you with the crucial data you need to make a well-informed choice. If your serious, chronic illness requires medical, not surgical intervention, ask your doctor, "How often do you see patients with my diagnosis?" Follow up by asking, "Are there any other alternative treatments I might consider that would work just as well or better?" From the response, you'll immediately learn if this physician is well qualified to care for you or whether your health can be improved with another treatment modality. You want to be treated by a healthcare provider who always works with people who have your illness. Forgive me for repeating myself to make a point, but my goal is to impress upon you the principal advantage of asking these questions. I get that these are tough questions and some people are very uncomfortable addressing their healthcare provider in this way. It's fine to be shy at a party, but in the doctor's office or the hospital your life and obviously your health depend on asking. It's truly necessary. When you're asking a physician to provide treatment that may be a critical step in returning you to good health, you'll want to have the optimum care available.

> After about a year Mr. B's tumor returned. Wisely, he chose a physician from an academic institution *who performed this procedure two hundred and fifty times a year.* This doctor was an outstanding choice for Mr. B. His surgery went well. Post-op recovery was quick and without incident. Unfortunately, by the time of his second surgery, the cancer had spread. He died about a year later.

I understand that finances and distance may limit physician and treatment choices for many people. What's more, you're not always in a life and death situation. I get that too. But, if there's any way to choose the most qualified/specialized person to care for you, the benefits outweigh the trip inconvenience and the cost. It's your life, right?

My great Uncle George had an uncommon cardiac abnormality that required a very rare and precise surgery. His local surgeon, Dr. X., advised him not to have the surgery at all. His doctor believed the chances of saving him with this surgery were very slim. But, Dr. X said, "If you'd like to get a second opinion (a wonderful suggestion), I can refer you to a surgeon who specializes in the type

of surgery you will need. Here's his contact information."
Bingo. (Some doctor's will even schedule the appointment
for you and, of course, provide a referral, if necessary.)
Without ego or hesitation, she graciously released her
patient to a more appropriate surgeon.

Uncle George: "Thank you for the referral. I'll contact her
immediately."

If a physician recommendation/referral was not forth-
coming from his local surgeon, he could have asked her
directly.

Uncle George again: "Can you recommend a doctor who
specializes in the type of surgery I need to consider? I
think it would make sense to seek a second opinion." (A
great question he was not too shy to ask.)

Dr. X: "Of course, George."

Remember: You always have options

Uncle George brought all his medical records and told his
story to surgeon number two who operated the following
week and likely saved his life. Well done, Uncle George,
Dr. X and surgeon number two.

It's also smart to do some research about the hospital
where you're having surgery, whether it's a simple outpatient procedure or a more complex operation.

Here are some important questions to ask:

- Have there been mostly good outcomes treating my illness here?
- Does this hospital share information about its safety and quality statistics?
- Does this facility accept my health insurance?
- What's the nurse to patient ratio?
- What's the incidence of MRSA in the hospital?

For more advice on being a hospital patient, read Dr. Marty Makary's book, *Unaccountable: What Hospitals Won't Tell You and How Transparency Can Revolutionize Health Care.*

Here are valuable questions to ask doctors and nurses, according to Dr. Makary:

- "Would you have your operation where you work?"
- "Does the teamwork here promote doing what's right for the patient?"
- "Do you feel comfortable speaking up when you have a safety concern?"
- "Are there other ways of treating this?"
- "What percent of these operations are done open vs. the minimally invasive way in the U.S.?"
- "What are the differences in complications rates for each?"
- "How many days will I be in the hospital if I have the surgery done one way or the other?"
- "Can I get a second opinion while I'm here in the hospital?"

You may also want to contact Citizens for Patient Safety, a non-profit organization, providing workshops for patients and healthcare professionals. Contact this group to learn more about its mission and how they may be able to provide even more education and direction for you, www.citizensforpatientsafety.org. You can also check out www.medicare.gov/hospitalcompare if you'd like to compare the performance of hospitals and read surveys as well. No computer? Call 1-800-MEDICARE for information. One more useful resource in your search to choose the safest hospital: Leapfrog—www.leapfroggroup.org.

In addition to all of these suggestions, don't hesitate to speak up if you have a question or a concern during your hospitalization. My mother, Florence Fendrich Segall, was the original "ask for what you need" and "lean in" woman many decades before Sheryl Sandberg. Shortly after being admitted into the hospital, she learned that her roommate's name was Shirley Siegel. You can see the problem straightaway. Florence quickly asked to be moved to another room to avoid any confusion given the similarities with her name and that of her roommate. In an attempt to reassure my mother, the hospital staff told her not to worry and that patient safety was their number one concern. Therefore, her request for a room change was deemed unnecessary and denied. The following day the phlebotomist mistakenly drew blood from my mother instead of Shirley. How did my mother know that? She checked the label on the vials. Blood work orders were for Shirley, not Florence. Guess what happened next? My mother was immediately moved to another room!

Hospitals work diligently to ensure they're treating the correct patient. If you've been either an inpatient or outpatient, you'll remember how many times you've been asked your name and birthdate regardless of the number of hospitalizations you've had. That being said, stay alert. The doctors, nurses, pharmacists, phlebotomists and anyone else who will be involved in your care are professionals, but mistakes happen. So, stay alert or have someone with you checking for any possible mistakes if you're not able to.

My mother had to "stay alert" when my father had his surgery many years ago. He had always been a quick healer but suddenly he began declining rapidly after surgery. The doctor kept ordering one x-ray after another to monitor any abscess my father might have at his surgical site. According to the hospital radiologist, there was no abscess. After several days of my mom's insistence that his post-op course was so unlike his normal, rapid healing while his doctor kept putting her off, my mom called a family relative who was a physician. He quickly had my father transferred to another well-respected hospital. When my dad was x-rayed at the new facility, a large, grapefruit sized abscess was easily and immediately visualized. Huh? A second surgical procedure was required to clean up the abscess. A healthier intestine was now created. How did the radiologist in the first hospital miss such an obvious abscess? Also, why didn't the first surgeon listen to my mother who knew that my father wasn't improving the way he normally would? This example is another excellent reminder to trust ourselves in any healthcare setting. Moreover, if possible, have a knowledgeable advocate at your side. Know that if your gut is telling you it ain't right (no pun attended), well then, pay attention. It doesn't make sense to wait until the situation worsens.

Personally, I'm grateful I've had the good fortune to be the daughter of Florence Fendrich Segall who confidently and consistently asked for what she needed long before women had the proverbial seat at the table. And to my father, Herman Segall, who always said, "The worst they can say is no." Thanks, mom and dad, for your example of persistence, perspective, self-confidence and conviction.

Always ask the doctor these **two absolutely essential questions:**

+ How many patients like me do you see a year?
+ If surgery has been suggested—How many of these surgical procedures do you perform a year?
  I know it's not easy, but you must ask these questions.

And, since you're asking questions, before finalizing any treatment, ask whether there are any alternative treatments that may be as effective as surgery?

Whether your health will be treated medically or surgically, **GET A SECOND OPINION.** Ask for a referral to a physician who cares for patients who have the same ailment as you.

By getting a second opinion, you may find a physician who has greater expertise in treating your ailment and who can suggest various treatment options that are available to you. It's always worth your time and effort to seek out a second opinion.

- Ask all your questions BEFORE you have surgery or a procedure.

- Query your doctor about how many of these surgeries/procedures he or she performs annually. Choose the doctor who does them most frequently.

- It's perfectly acceptable to ask whether there are non-surgical treatments to surgery.

- Find the doctor who specializes *only* in your serious healthcare problem.

It's essential to **speak up** about concerns. Your doctor won't know what concerns you, if you don't discuss everything that's on your mind.

CHAPTER 5
Re, Re, Respect!

Respect is the foundation of a mutually beneficial healthcare relationship—in truth, any relationship. I understand when physicians are very busy or not feeling well themselves, it can be a challenge for them to slow down, be polite and listen carefully. Bad days are universal. We've all had them. That being said, it becomes our responsibility to use the time we're spending with the doctor to get the most out of our visit as possible. Empowered patients can respectfully change the direction and tempo of an office visit. One way to achieve this is to provide all your healthcare information succinctly and clearly. (Review Chapter 2, Preparing for an Office)

This will be the most effective way to help your physician determine what your body is trying to say. But, if he or she is impatient, rude or disrespectful, it's okay to speak up. Actually, it's more than okay. It's necessary. Don't be intimidated if the doctor isn't listening, cuts you off or is condescending. Mutual respect is and always has been the cornerstone of a healthy, shared physician/patient relationship. It's also an essential starting point for becoming your own, best healthcare advocate.

Any healthcare professional, seasoned or less experienced, can become brusque or distracted. One young doctor just beginning his fellowship was so overwhelmed with a new computer system he couldn't take his eyes off the screen and look at me. After more than several minutes waiting patiently for him to look up, I asked him to give me his full attention instead of trying to figure out the new computer during my visit. I don't think he intended to be rude, but he should have spent time learning the computer program when he wasn't seeing patients! He was unaware his focus on the computer was detracting from the most valuable part of the patient/physician interaction—looking and listening to the patient. Ask healthcare professionals who have been practicing for some time and they will tell you the diagnostic clues they gather from a proper exam and listening to the patient is far more productive than the computer and test results. To his credit, this doctor apologized and directed his attention toward me. Hopefully, this friendly reminder will encourage him to forge a better connection with all patients and potentially improve his diagnostic skills.

Today, more than 70% of medical offices and hospitals use electronic health records, mostly referred to as EHR for meds, diagnostic codes, etc. These systems are quite efficient for doctors, but can leave the patients feeling as if they're not even in the room. The busy doctor who rolls her computer into the exam room and immediately begins entering your data is likely unaware you're feeling like an inanimate object. You might feel as if you have to shout, "Hello, I'm here!"

One night over dinner a friend commented that her doctor was far more focused on the computer than her. It so annoyed her she was ready to find another doctor who had a better person-to-person communication style. Instead, she wisely chose to advocate for herself by asking the doctor to look at her before entering the data into the computer. Her physician was truly surprised at how his behavior had impacted his patient. He immediately apologized. Future visits were markedly more communal and authentic, with the doctor's attention centered on his patient and her health concerns, not the data.

Patients, just like everyone else, feel valued and respected when they're heard and seen. Apart from that, the simple practice of observing and hearing patients is a powerful diagnostic tool. It's been said it's even more effective than all the high-tech equipment available today. Beyond that, creating rapport and mutual respect is a significant step toward improving or maintaining your good health with a physician who knows you and all your "health stuff" well.

Some physicians are employing scribes—assistants who are present in the exam room and enter patient information into a laptop. That way your physician can give you his or her undivided attention. Additionally, it allows the doctor more time without having to spend hour after hour entering notes about patients. Generally speaking, the majority of patients feel comfortable having one more person in the exam room with them when they're apprised of the scribe's purpose.

Besides Electronic Health Record issues, it's been my experience (having been a medical receptionist) that many healthcare offices overbook. Often, they're unaware of how much time is necessary for a patient's healthcare problem. It's best to ask for a longer appointment—instead of a ten-minute time slot—if you have a problem that you believe will need more time to address. And some people—like me—ask a lot of questions!

Several years ago, my own experience with an impatient, but very competent physician, was eye opening to say the least. After spending two hours in the waiting room, the doctor's staff told me politely the form they had mailed to me prior to the visit was the "old" one. "Please fill out the new one." No problem. Dr. W rushed into the exam room, obviously very busy and quite tense, and starting firing questions at me that required only a yes or no answer. His demeanor indicated he did not welcome me providing any further details about my health.

Since I had done what I always do—written down my questions in preparation for the visit (see Chapter 2, Preparing for an Office Visit)—I rose momentarily to get my iPhone to look at notes I had previously entered. I should have typed them out like I normally do and handed them to him. Oops! Dr. W's reaction assuming I would interrupt him: "When I am finished asking you questions I will *allow* you to ask me questions." I took a very deep breath and waited for him to complete his part of the patient interview. Then, we had what I like to call a *chat*. Me: "You will *allow* me to ask YOU questions? It would be a good idea to remove the word *allow* from any discussions you'll be having with your patients in the future. Creating rapport, mutual respect and listening to your patients actually will save you time and become more efficient. Plus, patient input has been proven to be a significant asset throughout the diagnostic process."

Dr. W: "I can't believe I said that. I'm so sorry." He then asked me if I was from New York! Of course, I am. For those of us who grew up in New York City, the real challenge would be to remain silent! Speaking up is never a problem. We both had a laugh. Still though, my point was not lost on him—treat your patients and everyone else with the respect they deserve. Maybe next time when he's rushed, over-scheduled and feeling impatient, he'll choose to take a breath, be more receptive and understanding of his patients' needs as well as his own.

Now that mutual respect has been established, future visits have been far more pleasant and productive. If you speak up and ask for what you need with your healthcare provider, you will be creating a mutually beneficial experience. Ask politely but do continue to ask until you've made it clear you're a patient who participates and advocates for your own healthcare.

Is it disrespectful when your physician is not listening to you? I think so. I usually give the doctor one more chance and make another appointment. If the second visit is just the same as the first—I believe I'm not being heard—I quickly leave and find another physician who is a far better listener. Physicians who listen to you are better diagnosticians. Plus, your recovery from your illness is generally quicker. Always make yourself heard. If your doctor isn't listening to you, find one who does. As I've said before, you have options.

My experience with a new obstetrician, who came highly recommended by my pediatrician (whose practice I left shortly thereafter) and several friends, had me literally sprinting out of his office after my second visit. Since this was my second child and I had previously worked for an ob-gyn practice for years, I had a pretty solid frame of reference. He began telling me when and I how I was going to deliver my son. There was no discussion. He never asked what delivery method I would prefer. On top of that, he used a simple, often incorrect test kit to check my blood type. He insisted my blood type was O positive which I knew was wrong. It's O negative. I shared my prior blood work and Rhogam experience. Still, he remained unconvinced. You could reasonably say that listening to his patients was not a skill he had perfected! Although I didn't know any other local obstetrician, I knew I would find another one who would hear me. I did a little research by both asking friends and checking out another obstetrical group practice (see Chapter 1—How Do I Find a Doctor?) which led me to a far better practice with a physician who listened to what I said. Thankfully, I chose another practice. My son was a breech presentation and a Cesarean Section was required to bring him safely into the world. I've always felt good about leaving a doctor whose style and skill I seriously questioned. Trust your gut. I'll say it again, *trust your gut.* If the "fit" isn't right with one doctor, if he or she doesn't respect your needs, doesn't hear you or worse, you question his or her competence, run as quickly as you can out of the office. DON'T BE INTIMIDATED. He or she is not the only game in town.

- Do you believe you're being heard? If not, courteously remind your physician why you're there.

- Empowered patients can improve the interaction between doctor and patient so your needs can be addressed more effectively.

- If your doctor is completely focused on typing notes on the computer screen, directly, but politely, suggest that he or she pay full attention and look at you.

- Again, speak up if your doctor is speaking at you, not with you.

CHAPTER 6

The Patience of the Patient

How much patience is enough and when is it time to move on? That's a question I've asked myself more than once and I'm pretty sure you may have as well.

This could not have been any truer than for my husband, Don. His employer at the time went bankrupt, we had an expensive home, his industry was in a downturn and I wasn't working at the time. Result? He was totally stressed out. As we've heard time and time again, stress is bad for your health. Shortly after he lost his job his skin began to peel for no apparent reason. Of course, there was a reason, but at the time, we had no clue what it was. The first dermatologist he saw never did a full body exam, but simply looked at one area of his body, told him he had eczema and prescribed a cream. The peeling grew worse. He saw another dermatologist who did a very cursory exam, (also examining only one part of his body), gave him some cortisone cream and sent him away. The peeling and rash continued to progress throughout his body. Two additional dermatologists in practice together both agreed he had psoriasis. They prescribed medication and additional treatments that further advanced the peeling and his rash. By this time, my poor husband was terribly uncomfortable with peeling skin from head to toe. Fortunately, he found another job that required a training period in Europe, but unfortunately, he felt and looked awful. And then, two other issues arose: his eyes became incredibly dry and *his skin had literally turned purple.*

That's when it happened. You know that little bell that goes off in your head when you're sure something isn't right? Well, that bell was ringing non-stop is my head. I kept thinking: "If this was psoriasis and he's being treated with the most current medications for psoriasis, why was he getting consistently worse?" I knew right then and there with the "bell" ringing 24/7, this was a **trust yourself moment.** I was sure research was going to lead me in the right direction. Since I was traveling with him, I sat down and began typing on a French keyboard—far different from the American one I was used to—and began running back and forth to the local shop to get the euros necessary to stay online. I was undeterred. My husband was suffering so and looked pretty awful as he started a new job. I knew I needed to act. First, I contacted The American Psoriasis Foundation, and asked which doctors in our local area back home were investigators (in a clinical trial) for new psoriasis medications. I got three names and picked one. Next I scheduled an appointment when we returned home. Lo and behold, dermatologist number five (really) took one look at Don's entire body and immediately exclaimed, "This is not psoriasis. I think I know what it is, but we'll need to do some blood work and several biopsies before we decide on an appropriate treatment." I wanted to jump up and kiss him, but I could sense he wasn't the type of doctor who would welcome a big kiss! Nonetheless, he literally saved my husband's life. It took close to three years for his skin to clear up and return his blood work to normal.

Every detail of this story is true and I've included them because I want to make this significant point: **Trust yourself.** If your health is getting worse, if your doctor is not thorough enough or if you don't feel as if you're being heard, it's time to find a different doctor. If your gut is telling you something is off, you're probably right. Trust what your body is telling you and act. You can always return to a doctor whom you've already seen, if after your research, you believe your healthcare professional is providing the best treatment available. Please encourage others to advocate for themselves too. All your friends, family, and neighbors need to hear you talk about advocating for improved healthcare. Your efforts can give them the confidence to speak up and seek out better care. Advocacy has the potential to change the course of an illness and save a life. Re-read the above story, if you have any doubts. My husband's illness would have been fatal, if not properly treated.

When I was a patient at The National Cancer Institute I remember looking at a large sign posted prominently in the hallway outside the treatment rooms. It read: SPEAK UP. Every letter urges you to ask for what you need. Here is what it looks like:

S: Speak up if you have questions or concerns. If you still don't understand, ask again. It's your body and you have the right to know.

P: Pay attention to the care you get. Always make sure you're getting the right treatments and medicine by the healthcare professionals. Don't assume anything.

E: Educate yourself about your illness. Learn about the medical tests you get and your treatment plan.

A: Ask a trusted family member or friend to be your advocate (advisor or supporter.) (More on this in another chapter.)

K: Know what medicines you take and why you take them. Medicine errors are the most common healthcare mistakes.

U: Use a hospital, clinic, surgery center, or other type of healthcare organization that has been carefully checked out. For example: The Joint Commission (a non-profit organization) visits hospitals to see if they are meeting its quality standards.

P: Participate in all decisions about your treatment. You are the center of the healthcare team.

Speaking up and seeking out the best care I could find was my goal when I was diagnosed with a serious, chronic illness. A very competent, kind oncologist was monitoring my blood work for a rare illness. In 2006, he said that it was time to begin treating me, not simply observe my worsening health. My first reaction: Whoa! Wait a minute! Because my oncologist was always open to listening to me we agreed that it made sense for me to be evaluated at a major healthcare center, The Mayo Clinic, with a physician who specialized in my illness. This is incredibly important!

I can't stress this enough: *Seek out an experienced physician who only treats patients with your healthcare problem. It's especially critical in rare or very complex illnesses.* It's smart and necessary. You need the professional who sees your problem every single day, not once in a while. When you choose a healthcare professional who has cared for many patients with your condition, he or she will be familiar with the most effective and most current treatments. What's more, the specialized, experienced doctor will know how to moderate and manage any potential side effects and problems that may arise from those treatments or the illness itself. What's most important: *Your ailment is far more likely to be diagnosed properly.* An incorrect diagnosis can lead to wasted time and worsening health. And as I'm sure you've heard, the wrong diagnosis can make you sicker or in the worst case, kill you.

So, how do you find out who is the best doctor to treat your particular illness? Re-read Chapter 1—How Do I Find a Doctor?

"Trust yourself.
You know more than you think you do."
–Dr. Benjamin Spock

Finding the balance between patience as a patient and frustration can be a tough call. How long do you wait? At what point do you lose faith and begin wondering if you're on the optimal path for your health? Basically, it comes back to that all-important message—trust yourself. Trust your gut feelings. We all hope for a miraculous recovery from a serious illness overnight. That would be wonderful, but it's not reasonable. Some illnesses require a bit of trial and error or experimentation to figure out how best to treat your problem. We'd love to think that doctors have all the answers to our health questions, but as skilled as they are, they're only human like the rest of us. But, if a prolonged period of time goes by and your condition doesn't improve or your illness is getting progressively worse, it's time to look elsewhere.

If you're worried or not sure what to do, call your healthcare provider and express your concerns. Don't be afraid to "bother" the doctor. That's what they're there for. It's better to call and find out it's nothing than to wait and watch your problems worsen. I had one of those "concerns" on a Friday. After beginning on a new medication, I noticed a rash. After several days the rash continued to spread to my back, my legs, my neck, etc. There was that little bell ringing in my head again. I'm thinking it's Friday. Better call now before the weekend. So, once again I chose to take my own advice and called my doctor. After examining me, he told me to immediately stop taking the medication. If I had waited through the weekend, the rash would probably have advanced even further. Why wait? Repeat that question to yourself over and over if you find yourself wondering whether you should call and be the annoying patient. Be the annoying patient. Be a P.I.A. (You can figure that one out yourself.) That's what Dr. A., whom I worked for years ago, called one woman. She asked a lot more questions than most other patients, but her concerns were addressed and she could then rest easy. Always be polite but be persistent. The squeaky wheel . . . You know that one.

If your body is repeatedly sending you a message that something doesn't feel right, listen to your body! The wisdom of your body is speaking to you.

SMART ADVICE

- If your health has not improved or has worsened for some time after multiple treatments you should consider choosing another healthcare provider who will look at your problem with "fresh eyes."

- Consider seeking special treatment from an academic/research university center. When doctors who specialize in your illness can't determine how best to treat your problem, the place to turn to is an academic center—a medical school. They're the most up-to-date when it comes to research and the newest techniques, procedures and medications. An academic center (university) can be the ideal place to treat your more complex problem.

- If your gut is telling you your treatment/physician is not right, your treatment or your current physician probably isn't the right one. Listen to it.

- Follow the recommendations featured in a large poster unmistakably displayed at The National Cancer Institute—SPEAK UP—where every letter emphasizes the importance of asking for what you need.

- Seek out the doctor who only treats patients with your type of illness. He or she will be the most knowledgeable and most familiar with the latest protocols and treatment options.

- Don't be afraid or concerned about "bothering" your physician with questions.

- Healthcare providers are educators as well as healers.

- Listen to your body. It's sending you messages you need to hear.

- Trust Yourself.

CHAPTER 7

Trusting Your Doctor ...but Not That Much

According to a Johns Hopkins study*, approximately 250,000 deaths annually were due to mistakes in the American healthcare system. Inpatients and outpatients were included. What caused these deaths? Communication breakdowns, diagnostic errors, poor judgment and/or inadequate skill. Take a look at what's on the list below:

The Wrong Diagnosis

A rare illness can be missed, but so can a more common one. Poor communication between healthcare professionals and patients, a narrow symptom focus (physicians focusing on a limited number of symptoms rather than the entire spectrum) or even gender/cultural biases may be contributing factors to a misdiagnosis. What's a patient to do? Make sure you understand what the doctor thinks your diagnosis is: ASK! If the physician is using medical terminology to explain your diagnosis, ask to have the word spelled out, write it down and do some research. You shouldn't try to read the entire text of *Grey's Anatomy* (the textbook, not the tv show)—but do understand the basics of your illness. You definitely need to ASK what those terms mean. Don't leave the doctor's office until you fully understand what your doctor is saying.

Next, what did your doctor rule out when he or she came up with a "working" diagnosis? ASK! In the book, *When Doctors Don't Listen*, the authors, Drs. Leana Wen and Joshua Kosowsky, consistently emphasized the importance of patients asking themselves if the diagnosis makes sense to them. Does it match your symptoms or not? Is your doctor telling you that you have the flu when you're there for a sprained ankle? If what he or she says doesn't make sense to you, repeat to your provider the reason for your visit in the first place. *Challenging your doctors respectfully is how you become an effective advocate for yourself.* When you get some test results that just don't seem reasonable or you don't understand the results, ASK. Don't just recycle or delete them haphazardly. Have you had the same test previously? If so, are these results dramatically different from a prior test for the same health issue? It's possible these are correct results, but they may also belong to someone else or be caused by a lab error. If you've kept your own healthcare records, you have an opportunity to compare the results. Additionally, if there's a patient portal you can access, it's easy to check on the results from your last test. Are the results very different? It's not a good idea to pretend all is well, have a glass of wine, and pick out what you'll be wearing to the party this weekend. Again, ask yourself if the test or the diagnosis makes sense to you. If not, repeat your misgivings to your healthcare provider. If you're still not satisfied with the answer, then it's time to get another opinion from a knowledgeable specialist.

Gloria, a nurse, who had a prior breast cancer experience, noticed a new area of concern on her breast. Her doctor kept telling her it was a dermatologic issue not cancer. After several weeks, the suspicious area became more enlarged and she insisted on a biopsy. Unfortunately, she was right. Years ago, my own mammogram showed some questionable spots. I was told to return in six months. Many women can relate to my experience and Gloria's, I'm sure. Since I come from a family with genetically predisposed breast cancer, I asked to have another radiologist read the films. Yes, he said, let's biopsy it. The outcome? Very, very early disease, excised by lumpectomy alone. I certainly understand that biopsies cause an undue amount of stress. I also understand that ruling out cancer is the primary objective. However, if it is cancer, treating it early may allow us to return to better health with a minimum amount of treatment.

Don't ignore your instincts and/or fail to acknowledge your own intellect. For those of us who are familiar with the book, *Winnie the Pooh*, I'm pretty sure you'll recall the wise words of Christopher Robin to Pooh:

"Promise me you'll always remember: You're braver than you believe, and stronger than you seem, and smarter than you think."

—A.A. Milne

If any parents are reading this now, you may recall the apprehension you felt with your first baby. I had no idea how to care for a baby. I was a stranger in a strange new land. When my daughter was about six months old, her pediatrician told me her fontanelles (the space between the bones in her head that gradually come together with time) were closing too early. Wait, what? There wasn't going to be enough room for her brain to grow normally. He scared me to death. He offered no reassurance. What do I do? My gut was speaking to me loud and clear. Uh oh—another bell ringer! It was saying "find another pediatrician now!" I did. Although her skull was maturing more quickly than most children of her age, the new pediatrician was willing to consider individual differences in her growth and development. He watched her closely. He was right to allow for her unique growth pattern. My daughter was then and is now fine. I was fortunate to have found a pediatrician who was smart, thorough, but not an alarmist. I always believed my kids and I were in capable hands and that was very reassuring. Again, trust your gut.

Confusion

It's not that healthcare professionals are often making really poor decisions, it's that some patients have more complex problems and sometimes, more than one medical problem. If that's the case, treatment choices can become challenging. A treatment for one illness may be incompatible with another. Since healthcare providers follow fairly specific guidelines for treating an illness, they need to dovetail multiple treatments safely and effectively.

So, what are patients supposed to do? We're not expected to be physicians, nurse practitioners or physician assistants, but we do need to stay alert or have a friend stay alert with us if we can't stay alert ourselves. That's when it becomes our responsibility to ASK for the details. Ask which guidelines your healthcare professional is following and make sure you understand them. Don't shy away from that question, although I understand you may need to take a deep breath and sit up straight before you can bring yourself to question their choices. Please do. Follow the three P's here: Be Patient, Pleasant and Persistent. What's more, you'll want to pay attention to your healthcare provider's reaction when you've gotten your courage up to ask the appropriate questions. If the doctor repeatedly resists treating your questions with respect, taking the time to answer them, you may want to begin the process of finding another healthcare provider. Remember you have choices.

Every time we moved, a new oncologist became part of my life. From Connecticut to Texas to Virginia, each oncologist watched my numbers rise. Every three months, I was anxious before and after I visited the doctor. Finally, in 2011, twelve years after my initial diagnosis, I asked my oncologist if he knew of any clinical trials at The National Cancer Institute I might be eligible to participate in. He turned his chair around, faced the computer and did a search. Yes, there was one! I enrolled in what's called a natural history study—one in which you have a significant abnormality, not a malignancy yet, but there's a good chance it will develop into one. About a year later I did have a blood cancer and became part of a clinical trial at The N.C.I. where I was treated for about three years. I will devote an entire chapter (Chapter 15) to the benefits, potential risks and what it's like to be a patient in a clinical trial.

But for now, my point is all about advocating for yourself. You must ask for what you need and most importantly, understand your options. How can you make an informed decision when you haven't been informed? I'm not questioning the competence of these physicians. They were all practicing quality medicine, but they were caring for many, many patients and had limited time to spend with each patient. In addition, they were following the standard of care suggested at the time. Nothing wrong with it, just not progressive or research oriented medicine. It's up to us as patients to question, take the time to research, and learn, as best we can what's going on in our bodies and to participate in any treatments that are recommended. *I can tell you that none of the oncologists I questioned as an empowered patient were the least bit defensive or threatened by my input.* Well, maybe by me, but not my input! In fact, when you collaborate with your physician or healthcare professional regarding treatment decisions, you become a partner in your care and share some of the responsibility. I've not met one doctor, either as a patient or as an oncology representative who didn't welcome that. Does your healthcare provider treat your input with respect? If not...

When I share the title of my book, the stories flow. They're often about themselves, relatives, or a good friend. All reiterate a simple point: I need to trust myself. To advocate. To be an empowered patient. Personally, when I've spoken up, most of the time I've had my needs met. I've felt reassured. Often, I've been right, but not always. It's okay for you and me to be wrong. At the very least you've used the opportunity to question, inquire and further explore what's going on in your body. It's easy to be intimidated in a healthcare setting. I know I've been. *Try not to allow your sense of intimidation to exceed your desire to quell those nagging concerns.*

Here's one more story to highlight my point. A young woman I sat next to on an airplane talked to me about her friend, 25-years-old, who had been bleeding between her monthly cycle. Her doctor kept minimizing her concerns. After several months of not being heard she went elsewhere and got the answer to her nagging question: Do I have uterine cancer? After a biopsy, she got the answer to her question. Yes, she did. After successful treatment by the second healthcare provider, she has been well. The bell ringing? The nagging voice? The feeling in your gut? These are all noises your body is creating to get your attention. Thank goodness this young woman listened to that voice and trusted herself. She put on her "big girl pants," took that deep breath and found her way to another doctor who took her very real concerns seriously. Her empowerment saved her. Why wait? Enough said.

As I've already written, everyone has a healthcare story about themselves, a family member or a friend. Many of these stories have nothing to do with cancer or other serious illnesses. Mostly they involve slip-ups, confusion or a forgotten order. They happen in some of the most prestigious hospitals and by some of the most esteemed healthcare professionals in the country. Whether you're old, young or anywhere in between, be confident in the presence of a healthcare provider. If you're respectful, polite and persistent, you're likely speaking with a professional who will hear your questions and answer you respectfully with the most current medical information available.

It's our responsibility as empowered patients to become active partners in our own healthcare. We can do much to help our healthcare professionals help us by providing clear, thorough information about our health and committing to a healthy lifestyle. In addition to many patient stories, I've listened to doctors share their stories as well. Patients arrive in their office with no comprehensive medical history, omitting huge chunks of particulars leaving the doctor at a total loss. Some patients don't know which medications they take, why they take them or how long they've been taking them. Other patients choose to go on eating cheeseburgers when their cholesterol is topping the charts and refuse to take an appropriate drug to treat it or begin an exercise regime. People smoke, drink, and generally abuse their bodies because they assume their doctor has a magic wand she can wave and make everything all better. That is, she can make them well without them having to change their poor habits. That would be great if it were true. But, of course, it's not! While I keep asking you to trust yourself and speak up, I'm also asking you (as you will note in Chapter 2—"Preparing for an Office Visit") to be a responsible patient, assemble your health records as completely and accurately as you can, write down your questions and be prepared to answer the healthcare providers' questions as thoroughly as you're able. I'm also suggesting you do your part in living a healthier lifestyle consisting of exercise, proper diet and avoiding stress. Your efforts will help your provider help you and hopefully, improve or maintain your health.

SMART ADVICE

- If you don't understand your diagnosis, ASK.

- If the doctor uses unfamiliar terms, ask for their spelling and definitions. Ask him/her to please write down those terms for you. Then, you can do some research when you get home.

- Know what illnesses your doctor has ruled out.

- Does the diagnosis match your symptoms?

- If you're still not satisfied with the diagnosis, get a second opinion.

- Ask about test results that don't seem reasonable. Compare the current results to earlier results.

- Don't ignore big differences/changes in your test results or your general health.

- Advocate for yourself and ask for what you need.

- Do your part in living a healthy lifestyle.

CHAPTER 8

Seek out and Connect with the Nurses

Nurses are very smart, capable and hard-working professionals. They're the go-to people for valuable clinical and drug information, guidance and support. Compassionate should be printed on their uniform! Several other "C" words also come to mind when I'm thinking about nurses: Clinically Capable, Competent and Credentialed. Nurses are the ones who support patients until they reach the finish line of their treatment. When I was a patient, I believed I could never adequately thank oncology nurses. They literally held my hand, laughed with me, and provided the medical information that the doctor was sometimes too busy to share. As I've often said, oncology nurses are angels who've floated down from heaven to get patients through some pretty rough times. I am forever grateful and humbled by their dedication and love.

Prior to my treatment when I was working as an oncology representative for a pharmaceutical company, I shared all clinical studies with nurses (the very same ones I'd shared with doctors) and the package inserts of prescription drugs. Of course, many of these drugs have significant side effects that need to be addressed. The nurses are the on-site side effect managers. And, believe me, they deal with a multitude of side effects that patients experience daily. Nurses are most often the ones who hear about side effects that patients are experiencing and forget to share (or are too embarrassed to share) with their doctors. Nurses are attentive listeners adept at answering many concerns patients have relating to their illness or their treatment. And, once those issues are cleared up they're more likely to stay on treatment (whatever type of treatment that may be—not necessarily a medication) and get well sooner. So, if you or someone you care about is receiving a complex treatment or even a far simpler one be sure to connect with a nurse. They're a valuable resource not to be overlooked.

Many people ask what nurse practitioners can do. Here's an explanation.

Healthcare and the provision of healthcare has changed immensely over the past fifty years, which is obvious, if you've been a patient in an outpatient clinic or hospital recently.

Over the same time period, the nursing profession has undergone significant changes. One of those positive changes is the inauguration of the professional nurse practitioner.

By definition, a nurse practitioner (NP) is a professional clinician who blends clinical expertise in diagnosing and treating health conditions with an added emphasis on disease prevention and health management. NPs bring a comprehensive perspective to health care. They are required to complete a master's or doctoral degree program and continue with advanced training beyond their initial registered nurse qualifications.

Once they are nationally certified, NP's can order tests, diagnose and treat acute/chronic health conditions, prescribe medications, and manage a patient's plan of care. Additionally, they are qualified counselors and educators guiding, supporting patients and their families along the path to improved health.

To be clear, the goal of nurse practitioners is not to replace physicians. They are part of the healthcare team—as are pharmacists, physicians and many other healthcare professionals whose goal is to help you feel your best. The approach of a nurse practitioner is holistic; he or she focuses on the health and well-being of the person as a whole. Promoting improved health, disease prevention, and directing patients toward smarter health and lifestyle choices is always their goal.

Ok, confession time. I am a nurse practitioner** who has spent a considerable amount of time over the past three years as a patient, basically on the other side of the stethoscope. This makes it a particularly uncomfortable place for me as a patient.

Nurse practitioners have played an integral role in the success of my care. Fortunately, an astute nurse practitioner identified an abnormality in my blood that led to a life-prolonging treatment. Many of my present clinic visits are spent with someone who listens to my complaints about medication side effects and encourages me to hang in there. It was a nurse practitioner who also helped me navigate the financial assistance application process enabling me to afford my very expensive medication.

Currently there are approximately 200,000 certified nurse practitioners in the United States. Chances are you will have the opportunity to meet with one throughout your healthcare journey. My hope is that you'll be open to including a nurse practitioner as a fundamental partner in your healthcare team.

**This excellent, informative blog that I've chosen to include in my book was written by my good friend and very knowledgeable, professional nurse practitioner, Kathy Carroll. Nurse practitioners are an incredibly valuable asset to our healthcare. So, the next time you're asked if you'll see the nurse practitioner, stop for a moment and reflect on the above explanation of their skills and training. Then you may say to yourself—why wait?

Not to be overlooked, PA's or physician assistants may be part of your healthcare team as well. They can also diagnose, create a treatment plan and write prescriptions.

They are healthcare professionals who have been educated for three years post their bachelor's degree and have passed a certification exam. Presently, there are 123,000 PA's in the U.S.

- ◆ Historically, credentialed PA's began in 1965 when a Duke physician—well aware of the need for additional medical personnel—was instrumental in creating the profession. The first PA's were corpsmen from The US Navy. Since that time PA's have undergone a medical school education, although somewhat abbreviated, and have worked with physicians in surgery, clinics, the VA, etc. in their role as healthcare professionals.

So, what's the difference between PA's and NP's? NP's need to choose a focus, that is, obstetrics, pediatrics, family medicine, etc. If they choose a different focus from their original choice, they would need to spend approximately 2,000 hours training in that discipline before they can change direction. PA's generally work in a surgical setting, although they can work in an outpatient setting as well. They work under the license of a physician, whereas NP's collaborate with physicians. PA's are not credentialed nurses. As mentioned above, PA's training is built on a medical school education and NP's are trained in the leading and current principles of nursing.

Both PA's and NP's are competent healthcare professionals who should be considered an integral part in returning you to good health.

- Nurses are competent, caring professionals who support you throughout any treatment you're having.

- Nurses are accomplished, patient, and attentive listeners. You should also share your questions and concerns with nurses to get the help you need.

- Nurses are knowledgeable and well-versed on medication, various illnesses and treatments.

- When you have questions about side effects or other problems with a treatment you're having, you've forgotten or are too embarrassed to share with your doctor, speak with a nurse.

- Take advantage of nurse practitioners and/or physician assistants. They're healthcare professionals with clinical knowledge and expertise who are able to diagnose and treat illness. In addition they focus on disease prevention.

- Nurse Practitioners can order tests, write prescriptions and create a plan of care. PA's can do so as well in both the US, the UK, and New Zealand.

- NP's focus on the whole person. They take a more holistic approach, guiding, directing and supporting patients to secure the help they need.

CHAPTER 9

Your Pharmacist Is Part of Your Healthcare Team

While we're trusting all of our healthcare professionals, (as we advocate for ourselves), we need to keep a close eye on our medications. To do so, you should consider asking your pharmacist, your healthcare provider and yourself the following questions:

- Has my medication been ordered?
- If I'm on a medication regularly prescribed, have I received it at the appropriate time to stay on the recommended dosing schedule?
- Is it possible the mail-order pharmacy forgot to order/ship it? If the provider did ship it, did it enclose the necessary and correct medication information?
- Has the recommended blood work been ordered

that may alter the dose or discontinue/change a medication?

If you're taking several different drugs, does each one of your physicians know what the others have been prescribing? You should let each doctor know the drugs you're taking now, what's changed, added or been eliminated. Again, you should help your doctor help you. He or she may not have the most current information about your prescriptions.

The most important question:
- Is this the correct drug for you, your kids, or your older relatives you may be caring for?

All of these questions are vital to our health. While pharmacists are ethical, smart, hard-working professionals, errors do occur. Quite a few of these errors are no fault of their own. For example, two different doctors order the same prescription and the patient takes double the dose necessary. This is not uncommon with the elderly or the very ill. I experienced this myself when visiting my elderly mother, checked her prescriptions and realized that two different doctors had prescribed the same cardiac medication and she took both medications.

In addition, the pharmacy may mistakenly insert the wrong patient information sheet in the little bag or in the mail. (This happened to me with my mail-order prescription. I'm sure my patient instructions didn't help the other patient at all!) Sometimes, your healthcare provider gets so busy that he or she forgets to order the appropriate blood work prior to writing a script which may mean your current dose is incorrect or ineffective. Although pharmacists routinely check for drug interactions, allergies, etc., slip-ups do happen. It's beneficial to check your scripts, as well as those of your parents, your kids and anyone else who is in your care before you leave the pharmacy. You may want to remind your partner to check his or her Rx too. Although they're not elderly or in your care, it's possible they're just not paying attention.

I know so many of us are in a major rush these days—work, gym, or posting on Facebook!—but, please do take a few moments and ask your pharmacist to help you insure that you're getting the right drug in the right dosage. Pharmacists are there to educate us, to answer our questions and review how best to use our medications. Let them. They're not just there to tell us which aisle the makeup is in! If you arrive at the pharmacy when there's a long line with patients waiting to pick up the prescriptions, have a seat, if you can. Wait until you have the opportunity to ask your questions and listen to the information the pharmacist has to share. Obviously, it's always best if you can have all your questions answered before you leave the pharmacy, but if you simply can't wait a while, call or better yet, return to the pharmacy to speak directly with the pharmacist. It's worth a few minutes of your time to gain the knowledge and reassurance she can provide. Additionally, it doesn't hurt to get to know your pharmacist and she know you in case an emergency or something unusual comes up. Pharmacists are well aware of the side effects your medication may present, or they can access that information quickly for you before you swallow that drug down. They can also let you know if your new medications will interact with the ones you're already on. That's especially important if your (kids, parents, loved ones) care includes several doctors who may be prescribing several different medications. Besides all the scary stuff pharmacists can protect us from, they can teach us how to apply and take medications in the way that's most beneficial to us. If we're not using meds appropriately, why even bother with them at all? You might as well spend your money at a casino.

Now, for a laugh from a true story. Years ago, I was working as a medical assistant for a group of obstetricians/gynecologists. A patient had been examined and she left the office with a prescription for vaginal suppositories. Several days went by. She called the office to say she wasn't getting any better. The suppositories hadn't cleared up her infection. The doctor asked how she was using them—always a very appropriate question, especially with a suppository. Her answer: "Well, I'm spreading the suppositories on crackers and eating them." Maybe that's why they didn't work! We all couldn't believe what we were hearing. While the doctor was on the phone we tried to be quiet and respectful. But, when he hung up, we couldn't stop laughing. I know it sounds like I'm making this up, but it's true. Some people would rather try to figure out how to take their medication in the most absurd way than ask the pharmacist how to use it. *Get over it and ask!*

In addition, you never know where you'll pick up a valuable medication tip. Case in point: While I was watching a Rachel Ray cooking show thinking I'd be getting some new kitchen mojo, a pharmacist was on the show demonstrating how to properly apply eyedrops. Who knew that there is a preferred way to apply eyedrops? Ask your pharmacist and you shall receive!

If your loved one is in a facility, hospital, nursing home, rehab, etc., you'll need to check with the nurses to make certain the patient is receiving the correct medications as ordered by the doctor. No one wants mistakes to happen, but they do. Older patients may not see/hear/understand/remember as well as they did years ago. I know from personal experience. My sister has been in a nursing home for years. Both my parents and grandparents were as well. Now that I have power of attorney (so necessary to establish for a family member or another trusted person) the nursing home often calls me when her dosage is adjusted, her prescriptions change or if she's ill. Although the nurses have many patients to care for, as long as you are the designated contact person, they will take the time to notify you of any changes in your family member's condition and her medication. In addition, it's not just the elderly who may have medication mishaps. Anyone who takes multiple medications, is seriously ill, in pain, and or confused is at risk for medication errors. Please ASK if you have questions about your medications. It's that important.

I'm willing to bet you're extremely careful before you give any medication to your children or even more worrisome, your grandchildren. Recently, while learning how to do video blogs, I recorded one about this topic.

My good friend and extraordinary meditation coach, Richa Badami (RichaBadami.com), and a very caring mother told me she always checks doses, proper medication and instructions for her kid's medications, but she literally flies out of the pharmacy when she's picking up a drug for herself. She never stops to check or ask questions for herself. Parents need to take their medication properly and stay healthy. Your health is every bit as important and probably more so than that of your family members. When the pharmacist asks if you have any questions about your own prescription, pause for a moment and say yes.

SMART ADVICE

+ Does the information enclosed with your script match the drug you've received? Both mail order and local pharmacies can make mistakes.

+ When you pick up a script, check to be sure it's for the appropriate drug for yourself or whomever you're getting it for (children, parents, your dog/cat, etc.) BEFORE leaving the pharmacy.

+ Ask questions about any side effects that you may have from a new drug or potential interactions with your current meds.

+ Proper use or application of a drug makes all the difference in efficacy. If the instructions aren't clear, ask if you must you take the drug with food or whether it's an external or internal cream, etc.

- Two different doctors prescribing the same or similar drug for you is obviously contraindicated and can be dangerous. If you consistently patronize the same pharmacy, the pharmacist can review a list of your prescriptions and see whether there are duplications. He may either contact you or your physician to double check the medication.

- If you have family members in a nursing home, stay in touch with their nurses. Your elderly or sick relatives may not remember if they have any drug sensitivities.

- While you're taking care of everyone else's medications, don't overlook checking on your own prescriptions. Ask your pharmacist about any concerns you have for medications you take.

- Don't spread suppositories on crackers!

CHAPTER 10

There's More Than One Way. We're All Different.

There's more than one way to get well. After many years as a pharmaceutical representative, national oncology trainer and now as a patient, I've heard many patients share their treatment choices. What I've learned is that there are many diverse paths to healing. Believe me, it doesn't need to be one way—my way or the highway journey. Each patient, armed with all the knowledge he or she can gather along with their supportive, very smart healthcare team and family will find their way—the way that works for him or her. In the past, I didn't always understand why people would choose complementary treatments instead of traditional ones or why they decided not to be treated at all. Now, I get why people make choices that others wouldn't make. Treatment choices remain at the discretion of the patients after they've very carefully considered all reasonable options.

Maybe you've had this problem for a lot longer than you'd like to admit and it just is not responding to the method of treatment you're currently receiving. Maybe this is a new problem. When I'm experiencing any of the above, I start by visiting a traditional physician or nurse practitioner. Their exam, along with any tests they order, often results in a *working diagnosis*—a place to begin figuring out what the healthcare problem is. It's not always that simple, however. Sure, if you have a cold or the flu, that's pretty straight forward. But, many of us show up with a problem that's more complex or with several, different symptoms. If that's the case, don't be surprised if it requires more patience—yours and that of your doctor's and possibly more than one doctor—to come up with an accurate diagnosis.

Guidance from my traditional healthcare professional is usually my first option. However, where do you begin if you're considering an alternative treatment method? How will you go about finding that information—Google research? Even before you begin "Googling," sit down quietly and do a little personal inventory—an internal review—basically, the prep I mentioned way back in Chapter 2, Preparing for an Office Visit.

Questions you may want to consider:

- Can you clearly identify the what, where and how of your problem?

- What have you already tried (other treatments/medication/surgery, etc.) to relieve your problem?

- How long has this been going on and what, if anything, you can recall, has precipitated this?

- And, here's a very BIG QUESTION to ask yourself: *What are my personal goals of treatment?*

For this particular health problem, you may also want to ask yourself: *"What can I control? What can't I control?"* Answering those big, pertinent questions will save you time, rule out what you've already tried, provide clarity and help steer you in the right treatment direction, so to speak.

Next begin researching your illness/problem and pay particular attention to what potential alternative treatment options may be available to improve your health. This could include complementary medicine—i.e., chiropractic care, acupuncture, supplements, a physical or mental exercise program, or simply observation.

Let me say quite clearly that I'm not advocating that you avoid traditional medicine. It's my own first chosen route, but I have, in the past, chosen acupuncture, physical therapy and counseling as *adjunctive treatments* for a nagging problem that traditional medicine has not been able to resolve. If you have a life-threatening health problem, however, selecting a curative treatment is most prudent. There are, though, many supportive healing modalities worth considering for less complex health problems that just might work well for you.

What may surprise you is that traditional physicians often support your choice to use complementary options for an ongoing problem. They want to see you get well and doctors realize there's more than one way to achieve good health.

Within that context, *it's essential to consider your own role in healing, what you're willing to do to get better, what your needs are and most importantly, your definition of healing.* Spend some time thinking about what you're willing to do to fix that knee, deal with your allergies, relieve that chronic back pain, etc. We all need to be very clear about what we want and what we're willing to do to get there. Sounds so simple, right? Actually, it's not. We are all very different, pretty darn complicated, and each of us has reasons for doing or not doing one thing or another to help us heal. Some of us want to be totally free of our existing problem no matter what it will take to get there. Surgery? Medication? Dedicated post-surgical, painful physical therapy and at-home exercise programs? A more restrictive diet? Quitting smoking, excessive alcohol use or the use of any destructive, recreational drugs? Can you commit to these choices? Figuring out where your head is at relative to your health issue is well worth the time spent. Once you're there, the road to your destination will often become clearer and easier to travel.

SMART ADVICE

+ When you're not getting better and considering alternative treatment, research all alternatives that relate directly to your problem.

- Do keep in mind there are diverse paths to healing with various treatment options. Be open to new experiences. Treatments are not a "one size fits all" approach.

- Most importantly, sit down with your very smart self and do some thinking. Begin asking yourself what you can control—better habits (food/exercise/stress relief) or cannot control (inherited issues)? And then ask the BIG question—what are YOU willing to do improve your health?

CHAPTER 11

Keeping Your Head Together Any Way You Can

Getting big, bad, scary health news is a blow, a major one. Literally, it feels like a punch in the gut. Your mind is reeling, your blood pressure is rising, and you wish you could find some solace, and walk away from your current, lousy situation. Receiving serious health news is terribly frightening. You begin to wonder if this is it and that you're going to die soon. Facing your own mortality is the most difficult, complex reality we all have to face at one time or another. Yet, no matter our age, most of us aren't prepared for that day. But, today, right now, here it is.

I have had the very same experience—the fear, shock and sadness. Therefore, I can tell you that I get it unequivocally. Any person diagnosed with cancer or another life-threatening illness gets it too. "I can't believe this is actually happening to me" is usually the thought that follows receiving the news. Total disbelief. After a few thousand, calming breaths (no kidding), my own reaction was never "why is this happening to me." It was "well, why the hell not me?" And later, "yes, it is definitely happening to me." It's an awful lot to take in. You're trying to get over the jarring, unhappy surprise when you realize you need *to do something, anything to get well, but what?* Besides learning exactly what your illness is, now you need to educate yourself about potential future tests, treatments, side effects, etc. That's an awful lot to deal with at once.

So, breathe . . . purposely, deeply, slowly, repeatedly and try to relax, even a little. Do whatever works for you: Meditate, reiki, prayer, exercise, open up a long overdue book, hobbies, support groups, time in nature, yoga poses, reading, hanging out with good friends and family, or a self-indulgent diversion like shopping—if you find that helpful. Check out the latest flick or anything that sounds like a bit of fun. Remember that bumper sticker . . . "I'd rather be fishing!" Well, whatever is your "thing," give it a shot. Whatever works is worth trying. To quote Oprah— "What I know for sure" and from Reina Weiner's personal experience—keeping your head together helps to lower stress and allows your body to focus on healing. Chill as much as you can any way you can.

I realize that readers of this book are going to be doing lots of research to become empowered patients. But, when you first hear your crummy news, it truly helps to take a break. As I'm sure you know, diversion from the momentary madness you're feeling can provide you with a clearer, more objective perspective. That's exactly what you need at the moment. You won't want to take a break because you want all the answers and the cure right now. I know. I felt the same way. Unfortunately, it's a process that takes time. And, unless you have an extremely acute or emergency type of illness, you can allow yourself to take a short break to get your head together. You'll be a far more effective advocate, if you step out of that frightening space for just a little bit.

I've accessed many of the previously mentioned options above for keeping my head together—or getting my head together in the first place—during my illness. Of course, I want the answers to my problem now, right now! Don't we all. But, take your walk, eat a great meal with friends, have a glass of wine, stretch and breathe. *The answers that are most appropriate for you will indeed show up. Know that. Have faith in your body, your healthcare team and the knowledge you're accruing toward healing yourself.*

SMART ADVICE

♦ There is a better way to respond to shocking and disappointing health news. The best response to the "holy S@t, I can't believe this is actually happening to me—I could die" feeling is to breathe. Breathe deeply again and again.

♦ Then, do whatever works for you—exercise, prayer, meditation, reading that book you started months ago, dinner with friends and if you'd like, a glass of wine or two. Most often, the answers you're looking for (treatment, etc.) take time to evolve. Use that time to relax while exercising the patience muscle. I know how hard it is. I've been there more than once.

+ Learn about your illness from reliable, professional, medical sources. Stay away from the scary and/ crazy stuff on the net.

+ Keep the faith as best you can.

CHAPTER 12

When You Can't Advocate for Yourself—the Grace of Allowing Others to Help You

The wonderful title of this chapter comes from my son, Daniel Weiner, and a mentor of his, Ram Das. Thanks to both of you for the words many of us need to read: Allow others to help you. I often need to remember that myself.

All things being equal, we'd like to be the ones who advocate for our own healthcare, by ourselves without anyone else's help. Ideally, we'd like to think we're able enough, have the time and the focus required to find out everything we need, and to get it done by ourselves. The operative word in the previous sentence is *ideally*. For so many reasons, the ideal is not always possible. Maybe you suddenly become seriously ill. Or, your computer skills are inadequate. Perhaps, your first language is not English. You may simply be so overwhelmed with your diagnosis that you sit in the doctor's office totally mute and just shake your head "yes" to whatever she tells you to do.

If the above descriptions apply to you, know that it's okay to accept help. In fact, it's more like mandatory than okay. Sit on your ego for a while and accept help graciously from anyone who offers. That includes offers of help to walk the dog, mow the grass, drive you to the doctor's office, take out the garbage or go to the supermarket for you. This is the time when you say, "Thank you, I appreciate your help sincerely," instead of the "No problem, I can do it all by myself" response. Before those "I can do it myself" words come out of your mouth, stop, take a breath and reconsider. Some offers, like the aforementioned ones, are time limited. If you don't accept assistance from people at the moment they offer, it may be one of those one-time only, this offer expires by Friday kind of thing. Really. While you're sitting on your ego, don't forget to stick your pride under your tuchas as well. Honestly, at this juncture, your ego, your pride, your stubborn, independent nature doesn't serve you well at all. I know because I'm writing about myself here. I don't love accepting help and I sincerely dislike asking for it. But, there are times when we truly need the kindness, generosity, and support of people who care about us. So, please, allow others to step up for you. Think of what you're doing for them. They'll be telling themselves what good people they are! Now, do you feel better?

Let's consider the nuts and bolts of allowing others to advocate or help you. Is there a person who might ease your way to wellness? Is there someone who has the time, expertise, connections or the knowledge within the healthcare community you may be overlooking? It could be someone you least expect. Let your circle of family and friends know that this kind of help is needed and welcome. You don't know what may come back to you.

A friend called me recently asking if I knew a researcher who could treat him for a life-threatening illness. I made some phone calls and came up with a name and number for him. And yes, it did make me feel like I had done something worthwhile. Do you find it impossible to take time off from work to do the research you'll need to get a handle on your illness? Or, are you simply confused about where to begin or how to advocate for yourself? Do you feel totally overwhelmed? I absolutely get it for all the above reasons. Let someone take your hand and show you the way.

To repeat: Be the vessel of grace and accept the help and support of others, whether you've asked for it or not. It's an essential element of healing. Why wait?

SMART ADVICE

- If you can't advocate for yourself now, accept the generous assistance of someone who can. Now is not the time for stubborn independence.

- Sit on your pride, your ego and say, "thank you" to any and all offers of help.

- Be the recipient, the vessel of grace and accept the support and love of others. It's an essential element of healing.

CHAPTER 13

The Power of Their Words for Good or Ill

Words are very powerful. The right ones can support our healing. But, those negative, sometimes thoughtless words can also compromise our healing in ways we're not aware of. Our healthcare providers and our healers can act in either of those ways unknowingly, likely with the best intentions. Yet, their words can add stress and negativity to an already stressful situation or they can encourage and sustain our healing. Choosing the right words is an art and a skill that physicians need to utilize on a daily basis. I know it can't be easy for them because they're human but those words are so very important to patients.

Years ago, I sought a second opinion from a world class, breast cancer surgeon. I wanted to know if I needed post lumpectomy radiation for a very early breast cancer.

Let me give you some of the backstory. At the time I was working as an oncology representative for a pharmaceutical company. I had daily meetings with medical oncologists, nurses, and pharmacists and got to know some radiation oncologists as well. I learned a great deal from them and was impressed by their professionalism and dedication to healing. After years of calling on them we had established comfortable, professional relationships. Therefore, when I questioned whether I needed radiation treatment after early, breast cancer surgery, the radiation oncologists literally opened their textbooks to me. I read. I learned. I researched the newest, most pertinent clinical trials. I researched the degree of risk my tumor presented based on the analysis of a respected pathologist. I even spoke directly with the Chairman of the National Surgical Breast and Bowel Project—the research arm for breast and gastrointestinal cancers. They're the ones who proved the effectiveness of breast conserving surgery—lumpectomy. When I called, the Chairman spoke to me for twenty minutes even though he didn't know me and I was not his patient.

Now, to the point: I believed I was well prepared to make an informed choice. Then came Dr. D's response to my question about post lumpectomy radiation: "If you don't have radiation, it will be the worst mistake you'll ever make in your life."! Boom! I felt like my head was going to explode. That was twenty years ago and I clearly remember every word he said. Talk about the power of words! His response shook me to my core. I had to take several very deep breaths and compose myself before I could even leave his office. Was I going to be responsible for making the worst mistake of my life as the esteemed

Dr. D. declared and not have radiation, or was I going to trust myself, and my research and choose not to have further treatment? That was a killer decision, I've got to say. I spent many days and nights reviewing, ruminating and obsessing over my choice, but finally I found peace with it. I was going to trust the learned opinions of many other radiation oncologists, pathologists, medical oncologists, surgeons and myself. No radiation treatment was my decision.

In the end, I kept my appointment with a radiation oncologist who looked at my pathology report and listened to me. His response: "I hear what you're saying. You're right. I could take your money, but there's no reason to. You don't need radiation or any further treatment." Another doctor I wanted to leap up and kiss! Those words—the "I hear what you're saying"—were the powerful, supportive words that gave me the affirmation I needed. I didn't have radiation. It's been two decades and I've not had a relapse in the same spot, which is, in the appropriate patient, what radiation post-lumpectomy prevents. It doesn't mean it will never come back in another spot on my breast. It can. But, for the last twenty years it has not relapsed right where it was originally. I feel very fortunate.

I'm not advocating you always ignore your doctor's advice. My purpose here is to emphasize how words from your healthcare provider can support you and help you feel safe during your healthcare journey or play a role in delaying your healing. Words are powerful and they matter.

I realize that I had open door access to quite a few doctors and their data. Many people don't. That said, everyone can do research, which is far more accessible online than it was back twenty years ago. Many doctors and healthcare professionals respond to email these days whether you're their patient or not. They may share their opinion with you—not always but it's worth asking your questions in an email—and be involved in your care. "The worst they can say is no!" Thank you, dad.

I keep hearing more stories from friends about their experiences with doctors whose words have not been well chosen. At the gym, one man was talking to someone about his recent visit to an ophthalmologist. The doctor said, "Well, I see you have cataracts. But, don't worry, you'll die before you need surgery!" How thoughtful. So very reassuring and sensitive—ha!

My good friend, Linda, was told by a resident physician her baby was now categorized as a "failure to thrive baby." The reason? He wasn't keeping up with the expected, "normal" weight gains for his age. He was too skinny. Of course, Linda being a new, worried mom went home and did her research. It said failure to thrive meant *death*! She asked the doctor what she should do. Feed him rice cereal. That's it—feed him rice cereal? You can imagine her shock and fear. As it turns out, this baby boy is now a healthy, skinny teenage boy. He is just like his slender father who will probably never have to worry about being overweight.

Again, the power of a physician's words can chill us to the bone while a softer, more thoughtful presentation can alter a patient's entire perception of a problem. Often, it's unlikely a doctor will know the exact trajectory of an abnormality or illness anyway. Even the most accomplished, respected physicians don't know exactly how your illness is going to progress. Every patient's path is different no matter how many people have the very same illness. We are all so unique. Unless there's a sudden, rapid change or an undeniable, significant, immediate health issue, it would be more reasonable for doctors to take your treatment plan one step at a time while monitoring you closely. I'm not a physician and don't claim to know close to what they know, but I have experienced the unnecessary, patient fear when presented, somewhat harshly, with the not-so-good news. I've been there. It can be incredibly frightening and the unintended stress can undermine your healing.

About seven years ago I was debating whether I should enter a cutting-edge clinical trial at The National Cancer Institute for a blood cancer, multiple myeloma. I heard many positive words. I discussed my potential choices with anyone who had an M.D. after their name (only kidding) and lots of friends/family. When I told my gynecologist that I felt very safe with the professionals at The NIH, she said, *Feeling safe is very powerful. Don't deny its importance.* That sentiment and those words stuck with me and soothed my questioning mind when I spoke with two medical oncologists who had been my doctors previously. "Don't do it. Absolutely not." That's what one physician said. Another one said, "Once you cross the Rubicon—meaning when you begin treatment—there's no turning back." He was right, by the way, when it came to basically non-stop treatment. But, he wasn't correct when it came to entering the trial. By the way, the Rubicon is a river in Italy crossed by Julius Caesar in 49 B.C. Don't be impressed that I know that. I had to look it up! But, the words of my gynecologist buoyed me, and I did enter the clinical trial, again showing the power of positive words. I participated in the trial because my illness had progressed and the question I had been ruminating over became moot, but the circumstances remained the same. Feeling safe and well cared for is very powerful. Don't underestimate it or negate it. Words that I've received throughout my time as a patient—when I needed all the supportive words I could hear—bolstered my morale, strengthened me, and supported me every step along the way.

I know there are times when you must hear the hard truth. There's no escaping it, and it can be excruciating to hear. It's also very hard for your healthcare providers to utter. I don't envy their responsibility. But, if those words can be shared honestly, with care and support, it does make the medicine go down a lot easier. A spoonful of sugar is always in order.

Most recently, I had an autologous stem cell transplant which means I've received my own stored cells. More about the process in another chapter. For now, obviously, the anticipation of such a challenging procedure was terrifying. I was looking for some sensitivity, some honesty along with some softness, from a social worker. She actually said, "That's a godawful, ghastly procedure to go through. I would only do it, if I had the best doctors in charge of my care." No kidding! As if I wasn't scared enough, those words coming from someone in the mental health community were far from helpful. Additionally, I had a nurse on the transplant floor tell me that the nausea I would experience during the transplant would be ten times worse than the nausea I had during pregnancy! Also very comforting. Turns out she was wrong. I had no appetite for months, but no nausea. Regardless of my transplant experience and its possible attendant side effects, support and soothing words from healthcare professionals go a long way in comforting our fears and providing a healing environment for our body. Words matter.

There are some hospitals currently requiring practicing physicians on staff to participate in a physician/patient communication skills workshop. Their goals are clear: training in reflective listening, empathy and how-to's for dealing with the patients whom the doctors consider difficult. Medical residents have communication skills built into their training, like the practicing docs, but throughout their training over a longer period of time. Both the experienced and the newer docs participate in role play. There's even an emphasis on the power of silence. Another meaningful communication challenge—simply listening. Less can be more, as you know. And, if everyone is talking, it's likely nobody is listening. I'm hoping that more and more hospitals will be facilitating communication workshops. They are beneficial to both patients and physicians.

- Words can heal and support us as we go through health challenges. Negative, fear-inducing words may delay our healing and add unnecessary stress when we're facing an already frightening health issue.

- Although many doctors understand the significance of their words, rushed, overworked physicians may not be aware of how powerful their dismissive and pessimistic words can be. Patients take their physician's words home and live with them for good or ill.

- Patient/physician role play seminars to improve reflective listening skills and empathy are being required in more hospitals around the country. This is an excellent example of medicine moving forward in a better direction.

CHAPTER 14

The Three P's—Patient, Pleasant and Persistent

After all this writing about participating in your care, asking for what you need, creating mutual respect, etc., did I even mention how to go about it? No! Well, here are the three P's—my go to strategies for making it happen.

First and always **be patient.** I always want to believe that most people working in a doctor's office—the receptionist, the medical assistant, the nurse, the nurse practitioner, or doctor—are doing the best they can. I try to remember there are patients who have more immediate needs than I do. There are patients who arrive late for their appointment, emergency patients who need to be seen ASAP, patients with serious concerns who require more time than the doctor anticipated, insurance issues, possible procedure scheduling, pharmacy calls, and on and on. I understand. Although my issue is my first priority, it's often not a priority in the doctor's office. Therefore, nurturing and focusing on patience will surely be an asset. If your behavior indicates you're annoyed and your words support your impatience, you may find you're waiting even longer. No one wants to be spoken to rudely. Asking politely when you may be called, if you've been waiting for quite some time, is a fair question. Don't go up to the receptionist every five minutes and ask when it's your turn. But if you notice many patients being taken in before you, then it's appropriate to ask the question.

In addition, patience may be required if you're waiting for test results, or a call back from your doctor's office with an answer to your question, or if a prescription has been ordered. Do check back as orders can be misplaced and test results can be waylaid as well. Or, the test results may be on the doctor's desk and she just hasn't gotten to it, or the lab is taking longer than expected. Patience, patience, patience.

Be Pleasant. I can't say that often enough. My father used to say you catch more bees with honey than with vinegar. That's still true to this day. At least, start out pleasant! You always get much more mileage when you treat others with respect and kindness. Besides, you're a thoughtful person. Kindness comes naturally, right? Well, even if you've had an awful day, pause and think of how you'd like to be treated when you are having a less than perfect day. I can remember being a medical receptionist and being the recipient of someone's anger. That angry tactic definitely won't get you in to see your healthcare professional any sooner. For that reason alone, it's best to smile, be polite and patient.

And lastly, **be Persistent.** That doesn't mean to lose your patience or your pleasant demeanor. It does mean don't give up. If your questions are not being answered, your prescription doesn't get filled, no one is getting back to you with test results, keep calling, emailing, texting and asking. As I mentioned, your results or records may have gotten lost, misfiled and somehow mistaken for someone else's results. It happens, more often than you'd probably like to think. As a result, you certainly need to be persistent. Ask, ask, and then ask again. It's possible that your healthcare provider never got your message or doesn't know you have a request. Here's what I do: If I haven't heard back from my doctor's office after a day or two, I get back in touch. The number of times that I've re-written an email or called again are many, but that hasn't stopped me. I just keep on asking until I get what I need. It may be after a long, holiday weekend or vacation and your doctor's office is overwhelmed with requests. It may be that your request or test results is under a pile of papers on your doctor's desk. I'm not a believer in the "no news is good news" concept. Trying to pretend a problem doesn't exist is not smart and it doesn't make it go away. Also, delays in addressing your healthcare problem may make it more difficult to treat in the future. Persist until you get what you need.

Be Patient, Pleasant and Persistent. It works in a medical office and just about everywhere else.

◆ It's all about the three P's—Be Patient, Pleasant and Persistent—to get things done.

◆ Be Patient while staying vigilant when "stuff" happens in your doctor's office or hospital. Emergencies, unexpected problems requiring lengthy patient visits can throw your doctor's schedule off. Bear in mind that patient could be you one day.

◆ Be Pleasant. Begin conversations with your healthcare provider, nurse or pharmacist in a pleasant manner. You definitely "catch more bees with honey than vinegar."

◆ Be Persistent—If you've been waiting for test results, a prescription, or aren't getting your questions answered, don't assume that everything is well. Ask courteously until you get what you need, but don't give up.

CHAPTER 15

What Is a Clinical Trial?

What is a clinical trial? Briefly, it's an extremely comprehensive, scientific research study that involves human subjects (studies that involved animals are pre-clinical) and analyzes treatments that have the potential to treat or cure illness. Because clinical trials are scientific studies, patients are very carefully monitored. The study is strictly controlled and regulated in order to ensure it is scientifically valid. The goal of each study is to ensure that this newer treatment is safe, effective, tolerable and better than current treatments available presently (considered standard of care) before it becomes available to the public.

Clinical trials go through multiple approval phases, ethics boards and regulatory agencies with research scientists, doctors, nurses and lawyers before they are approved to enroll patients.

Each phase of a clinical trial has a specific objective. A *phase I trial* is designed to learn the *MTD—maximum tolerated dose of a drug or drugs*—a dose that is safe and tolerable. Patients who participate in phase I trials are generally those who have already been treated with a host of different treatments without improvement to their health.

After phase I is complete the scientific study moves on to a *phase II trial*. Each phase has a new objective with different participants. The goal of a phase II trial is to learn if a new drug works, or more appropriately, *if a patient's illness responds well to this new drug or combination of drugs.*

Lastly, a *phase III clinical trial compares standard of care treatment to the new treatment.* Its goal is to determine whether the new treatment is any more effective than the earlier one. In cancer clinical trials, phase III trials also evaluate (have an *endpoint*/goal of) *survival*. The question the study is designed to answer: Does this new treatment keep patients alive longer? Also, does it provide patients with a longer time to disease progression? Additionally, phase III trials are randomized. What the heck is *randomization? It's the process used to select patients randomly to be assigned to one of two arms (groups) of the trial.* Most often, neither the researcher or doctor knows if a patient is receiving the new treatment or the older standard of care. That's the true definition of a *double-blind* study. If you're wondering what happens when patients on one "arm" of the trial are responding much better than those on the other arm, the trial is quickly unblinded or opened and every patient is then given the more effective treatment. Ethics requires that.

All of the above has to happen before a new drug application is submitted to the Food and Drug Administration for approval—which then goes through the lengthy process of approval. It's not unusual for a drug to take about fifteen years from the day that someone has a brainstorm about a new treatment and it finally gets approved for use by the public. Why is this process so long? There's an almost infinite number of questions about safety and efficacy that must be addressed from a scientific point of view, plus tons of approvals throughout the process. What's important to keep in mind too is that many drugs never make it to market because they just don't work any better than what is currently available or they're not safe. Lots of time and money is often spent on trials that don't yield any new therapies.

Who pays for clinical trials? Pharmaceutical and biotech companies provide funding for clinical trials within a carefully regulated and collaborative process. Academic researchers and scientists from the drug companies collaborate under very strict guidelines. Congress also allocates money for research to The National Institutes of Health and some charitable organizations provide research grants as well. When you're complaining about paying your taxes it's a good idea to remember that some of your money is going toward research which moves medicine forward benefiting us all. Thankfully, it's not just pharma picking up the entire tab.

Are you wondering who is looking over the shoulder of both researchers and pharma to keep them "legit?" The FDA and the internal review board of the clinical trial are doing plenty of looking at the trial and all aspects of it.

Plus, the pharmaceutical company supporting the trial is being reviewed on a regular basis—both within their own company and the FDA/internal review board of the trial—to be sure everyone is following the protocol and making sure the study is adhering to all the guidelines. Due to all the extensive oversight it's almost impossible to bias the study in favor of pharmaceutical companies. The reputation of an institution, the integrity of the researchers and the validity of the scientific data of the clinical trial all depend on its unbiased accuracy. And that doesn't even address how the results of the clinical trial will affect patients in the future. I've talked with many researchers throughout my career in pharma and as a participant in several different clinical trials. I know how determined they are every day to find new answers to old problems. The rigid processes, the length of time involved, the efforts to encourage patients to participate in clinical trials combined with all the frustrations and failures researchers often face have given me nothing but the greatest respect for researchers trying to and hoping to advance medicine.

Since I've explained the development, the oversight, the phases and the regulated safety of clinical trials here's my take on what it's like to be a patient in a clinical trial. I've participated in four.

You know what most people say when they learn I've volunteered to participate in a clinical trial? "Aren't you a guinea pig when you're in one of *those*?" If people don't say "guinea pig" that's definitely what they're thinking. Besides, many people asked my husband why he would "allow" me to be included in a trial. There's so much fear and misunderstanding about what a clinical trial is and what's it's like to participate in one.

Here are a few questions people frequently ask:

+ "Are they using a placebo/sugar pill?" Administering a placebo is extremely rare in a clinical trial for cancer and occurs only in a Phase 3 or 4 trial. In earlier level trials using a placebo would be unethical. The goal of clinical trials is to improve your health not put you at greater risk.

+ *"Can I drop out of the trial?" Yes. You can drop out of a clinical trial at any time and for any reason.* Of course, if your illness progresses while you're on the trial, you will need to leave the trial. Your physician will guide you to another treatment that's appropriate for you.

+ "Is it scary?" Yes. Cancer itself is pretty darn scary no matter where you go for treatment. For me personally and I'm sure with all patients, our goal has always been to receive the best treatment available. But, even more importantly, when you enroll in a clinical trial you have the opportunity to be part of the big picture, that is, a potential cure. Yes, it may help you. That's true. Far more significant, though, is the potential that clinical trials may provide new treatments for patients who may follow you in the future with the same illness.

And, as you already know, people have to give their consent to participate. What can you or someone else you love do if your health is threatened? ASK YOUR DOCTOR ABOUT A CLINICAL TRIAL. It's really that simple. Your physician can research available trials on the computer pretty quickly. If there is a trial for your illness, please consider participating. When I've spoken with many other clinical study participants here's what they've said, "If my participation in a trial helps other patients, I'm happy to play a small part in curing them or at the least, improving their quality of life." Hearing the altruism of patients while they're going through their own, significant health issues is heartwarming. Additionally, it also takes a little bit of courage and plenty of empathy to choose a trial. It's always reaffirming to learn there are still lots of great humans left on the planet.

YOU ARE NOT A GUINEA PIG! Trials are very carefully monitored by researchers, lawyers, ethicists, academic centers (if they're involved) and the pharmaceutical company that may be sponsoring the trial, the FDA, etc., etc. When I participated in my second clinical trial (my first trial was strictly observational) the number of people who asked my husband why he would let me be part of the trial was truly remarkable. There's so much fear and misinformation surrounding trials which is unfounded. Years ago, there were some unethical medical studies. You may have heard about The Tuskegee Study of Untreated Syphilis in the Negro Male **(conducted between 1932 and 1972)** which surely contributed to the fear that many African American patients have volunteering for a trial even today.

The first clinical trial I participated in was at the National Cancer Institute, part of the National Institutes of Health, in Bethesda, Maryland—a group of twenty-seven different research centers organized by health issue. (By the way, the N.I.H. is the biggest research institution in the world not just in the U.S., but in the world.) Plus, I've participated in two more at The National Cancer Institute. I've also participated in one at Memorial Sloan Kettering Cancer Center in New York City. During all four trials I felt safe, well cared for and believed I was receiving the most cutting-edge treatment available at the moment. To that point, the treatment I had in 2012 is still not approved for newly diagnosed patients and probably won't be for another several years. That in itself was a significant motivator for me to join the trial. Additionally, I believe strongly in research as the only way to advance medicine for the benefit of future patients. On the other hand, as a clinical trial participant, I did have more blood work, more bone marrow biopsies and closer monitoring than I would have had if I had not been in a trial. I knew that going in. All patients in clinical studies are well informed regarding the tests and exams they will be volunteering for as trial participants. There are no surprises. Being followed so closely was definitely in my best interest and honestly, I was grateful for that. Any problems that arose could be quickly addressed.

Would I enter another trial? A definite YES! As a matter of fact, I tried to enter trial five recently, but I was ineligible. In order to ensure scientific integrity, trials are quite rigid in their design. Often, patients who would like to participate don't meet the qualifications and are not accepted. Being rejected from a trial is frustrating and disappointing. I know that's how I felt when it happened to me. But, although you're not eligible for a particular trial, you may be eligible for another one in the future. New trials are constantly being formulated. As long as there's funding available (and an adequate number of patients willing to participate) there will be valuable discoveries waiting for us all on the horizon.

Did you know that only 3–5% of all cancer patients— out of about 3 million annually—participate in clinical trials! That number is so incredibly small— certainly not enough to create reliable data—which then slows medical advances and research for new treatments down to a crawl. Small trial numbers, unfortunately, don't have the "bang" as ones with large cohorts of patients. Ask any scientist. They don't consider the data as reliable from a study with a minimal number of participants.

Of course, there are trials for many different illnesses, not only cancer. Each trial plays an essential role in improved treatments, better quality of life and hopefully, longer survival rate. If you've got a problem that has doctors scratching their heads about, using the same treatments they've tried for years without success ASK IF THERE'S A CLINICAL TRIAL FOR WHICH YOU MIGHT BE ELIGIBLE. No one suggested a trial to me until I asked!

ASK! Doctors get so busy with all their responsibilities and often, way too many patients, they may forget to ask you if you'd consider being part of a clinical trial. Don't be shy. Speak up and ASK.

If after asking your doctor to help you search for a clinical trial and he/she is unable to, please be sure to google a support organization for your illness. Contact them. They will likely be able to do a clinical trials search or direct you to another organization who can do the search all free of charge. Consider searching clinicaltrials.gov with your diagnosis. It's a more arduous and overwhelming search so be sure you have a clear definition of your diagnosis. You may need some help. One more way to find a trial is to contact an academic institution and ask for someone who can assist you in doing a clinical trials search as long as you know your diagnosis. It make take some doing so please be patient.

There are many trials groups and academic centers throughout the country that offer clinical trials. Medications are free of charge. Some trials also cover tests and exams, even travel. All the details and relevant information is available to you before you agree to participate in the trial. Do ask about the particulars, if you're considering participating. In addition, there are charitable foundations that may be able to help you financially, whether you're in a clinical trial or not. A support group which helps people with your specific illness can advise you and may refer you to other groups or foundations. For more about financial assistance and support groups, read Chapter 17.

Before you agree to participate in a clinical trial here are some questions to ask of the researchers:

1. What are you (researchers) trying to learn from this study?

2. What will I need to do?

3. Will the study be of benefit to me or others?

4. What are the risks? And, what are the chances that there will be risks?

5. What side effects might I experience?

6. What will my time commitment be?

7. Are there other inconvenient aspects of the trial I should know about?

8. Can I discuss my participation in the study with my family and friends?

9. Do I truly want to participate in the study? (Ask yourself this question)

10. Are there consequences, if I decide not to participate in the study?

11. How soon do I need to let you know one way or the other?

12. After the initial study, will there be further follow up?

After you've had time to process all the answers you've gotten from the above questions, you will be ready to make your decision. If your answer is "yes" to entering the trial, then the first step is to sign the consent form. You will receive a "consent to participate in a clinical research study" form that clearly explains all aspects of the study. A healthcare professional will go over the protocol (regimen) and answer any additional questions you may have. You will have a period of time to consider whether or not you want to consent to the trial. There will not be any pressure to participate. In addition, you may choose to leave the trial at any time after you sign the consent form, no matter where you are in the trials process. If you decide to leave the clinical trial because you can't tolerate the side effects of treatment, you don't have easily available transportation, you have to take off from work, or your trial participation complicates your family responsibilities, or for any number of reasons, you will then return to the doctor who previously cared for you.

Clinical trials can be beneficial for you as well as other patients who will follow you. But, I urge you to ask as many questions as you need to before making your decision to participate in one. Please remember to ask about a million questions until you decide one way or the other.

- A clinical trial is a scientific, research study that functions within a strict protocol that's extremely well controlled with human subjects. The goal is to search for new treatments to improve the health of patients and possibly find a cure to illness.

- Trials are organized in three phases each with a specific endpoint or goal.

- Trials are meticulously designed and painstakingly monitored. Concerned about who's keeping the trial legit? Internal review boards within the F.D.A., academic institutions, The N.I.H., principal investigators and pharmaceutical companies, if they are involved, are attentively ensuring that the trial is adhering to its goals and the proper collection of data. Researchers, lawyers, and ethicists from all participating institutions work to ensure the safety and scientific validity of the clinical trial. Pharmaceutical companies cannot bias the trial results in their favor because of the uncompromising structure of the trial and the continuous oversight.

- Who pays for a trial? The National Institute of Health (our taxes), pharmaceutical companies and grants to individual researchers, or a combination thereof cover the costs.

- There is a great deal more oversight of treatments in a clinical trial than you would receive in traditional hospitals or treatment centers because of the need to maintain the integrity of a clinical trial. How do I know this? I've been a patient in four clinical trials.

- There are no "guinea pigs." The emphasis is always on the patient's safety.

- If a trial hasn't been offered to you, ASK your doctor to help you find an appropriate one. If he cannot find one for you, do your own research by going to a non-profit support organization focused on your illness, a foundation, search clinicaltrials.gov by putting in your diagnosis, or contact an academic institution (with a medical school), and ASK to be referred to someone who can help you search for a clinical trial.

- Clinical trials are not just for cancer patients. There are many trials seeking answers to various chronic illnesses. ASK your doctor.

- Review all the questions patients should ask before they enter a trial.

CHAPTER 16

Keeping Accurate and Up-To-Date Medical Records.

Let's say your doctor has requested a certain test, procedure or written a new prescription. Has another physician ordered that test or the same drug?

If this has happened, then speak up! Don't be shy. My favorite word throughout this book and I hope will stay with you is this one word: ASK! Learn why this test is being ordered and how the results may impact your diagnosis and future treatment. Be sure you're clear about the reasons and whether they make sense to you. Unless it's been determined that an immediate test or procedure is necessary for your health, consider whether you'll choose to have the test right now or defer it to a later date.

A panoramic, dental x-ray had been ordered for me as part of a standard, dental work-up. Having kept a record of prior x-rays I was able to politely and clearly decline the x-ray because my records indicated I had one six months earlier. If I hadn't been aware of and kept my medical and dental records, I would have had to have additional, unnecessary x-rays. This wasn't an invasive procedure but there wasn't any reason to duplicate what was already done. I still have the same healthy teeth as I did six months ago!

Nowadays there are patient portals—an online record of your test results, your physician's notes, upcoming appointments and insurance/billing information. But, as helpful as these portals are, there is no physical evidence of test results. In other words, the films (x-rays), the MRI results on a disc, the CT scan or your pathology slides (if you've had a biopsy) are not available to you unless you ask for them. In order to get them you will need to provide a written request to the radiology department or the pathology department directly. Don't leave the office, hospital, outpatient clinic, etc., without those results in hand. I may sound like the credit card commercial! But, it's true. Other than the biopsy slides, which can take time to copy, you can pick up the CDs of MRIs and x-rays at the time of your visit. Having that actual, essential piece of your healthcare history will likely determine the direction(s) of any future treatment you may need. It's *not* the written report you and your doctor will receive later, but the actual physical, tangible, results of your tests. If you're seeking a second opinion, seeing a specialist, if surgery is suggested or you're moving to another community, those actual records are exactly what the new doctor will want to review. Most physicians will want to look at those results and come up with their own diagnosis independent of the input of other physicians.

Trying to get the MRI or the CT disc, the films, and the slides later on is much more difficult than asking for them at the time the test is being done. You will need to call, email, text someone who will search for the records for you. Then you'll probably need to sign a release, once the films or slides are located. Most records are stored for a period of time but as time passes, it may be more difficult to get them. They can get lost, damaged, misplaced, misfiled or accidentally discarded. In other words, it's a big pain trying to get your "stuff" next week, next month or two years from now. Often, the responsibility falls on the medical receptionist or nurse to locate your records and have them forwarded to the appropriate physician. Knowing whom to contact and how to contact them can also be an issue. It's not that people don't want to help you. They do. But, when other people have to go searching for your records they may not have all the detailed information they need to locate your records. It makes life and record retrieval so much more complicated and far less efficient. Simply put: More people = more time and confusion. Again, the best, most efficient manner to pick up your physical medical records is to request them at the time of your test. And, sorry to be redundant but, after asking for your "stuff," make sure you take everything home with you at that time. You may need to wait a while until the staff can get you what you need, especially if it's a very busy facility. It's worth the wait. Read a book, play a game on your iPhone, meditate or daydream, but don't leave. You will save yourself and your healthcare providers time, energy and frustration if you can be patient and chill until you get what you need.

I recently spoke with a nurse, who is a friend of mine. She emphasized how much of her time is spent searching for patient records in an outpatient unit. Obviously, a physician wouldn't proceed with any invasive procedure or even a non-invasive procedure without first obtaining all the pertinent previous data. Consequently, the procedure is held up. And as for the nurse's time, she could then devote more time listening to you, supporting you and sharing helpful medical information with you instead of sending emails, texts and waiting on hold to speak with someone who can locate your records and get them to her. She told me that she spends more of her time chasing medical records for patients than anything else. That's certainly not the best use of a medical professional's expertise!

I know you get my point by now. Please be sure to request your records and leave with them in your hot, little hands after your appointment. And, do remember to bring them with you to your upcoming appointment. Put a reminder in your phone, a string around your finger or put your records in your car the day before your appointment. Why do I stress these little reminders? Probably, because I've gathered all my records together and promptly left them home! It doesn't do much good, if you don't have them with you.

- By keeping an accurate, up-to-date history of your medical records, you can avoid unnecessary repetition of medical tests. Keep these records in an easily accessible place so you don't spend time searching your kitchen drawer, medicine cabinet and who knows where else.

- If a test or prescription is ordered and you don't understand the reasoning behind it, one more time: ASK! You may just save yourself the duplication of a drug or a test by having up-to-date medical records.

- Although patient portals are an efficient way to stay in touch with your healthcare provider, you can't get the actual, MRIs, x-rays or biopsy slides through the portal. You'll need to request those directly from the facility where you had the procedure.

- When do you need the actual MRI, CD, or biopsy slides not the written report? If you're getting a second opinion before surgery, visiting a specialist whether you've seen him or her previously or moving to a new area, the physical data is relevant. Always take those records with you—the CD's—at the time of your test and be sure to take them home with you after the physician has reviewed them.

- The quickest way to get the physical results of your tests is to ask for those results at the time you've had the test. CD's are relatively easy to get. The biopsy slides will have to be copied and that can take some time. Additionally, you may be under anesthesia when you've had a biopsy. That's probably not the appropriate time to talk, but when you're up and about, ask for a copy of your slides.

- Trying to get the CD of your results a while after you've had the test—not the day of—will require the help of others and will take some time. That's why it is always preferable to get them before you leave the facility.

- Nurses and office staff who have your records will spend more time with you, answering questions, if they don't have to spend time retrieving your records from other physicians.

CHAPTER 17
Financial Aid

Getting sick is too darn expensive. That sounds pretty callous, but it's true. You need money to get well. Either you'll be paying for your insurance premiums or if you don't have insurance, paying for treatments out of your pocket. Somehow, the bill has to get paid. I know how expensive new, targeted, cutting edge treatments can be. I also know that many healthcare professionals don't know how much the drugs that they're prescribing cost. It's not that they don't care. They do. But the physicians have a lot on their plate from all their interaction with patients to today's increasing demands of the business of medicine. That said, it's up to us patients to ask for what we need! (Sound familiar?).

In this chapter, I'll be explaining some of the costs of keeping you healthy and how you can lessen some of these expenses.

If your doctor is ordering a prescription medicine for you, ask if there's a drug a that's bio-equivalent (she'll be impressed with that word!) that's less expensive. Of course, the alternative needs to be as active and effective as the brand; otherwise you might as well eat gummy bears. But, if there is an appropriate drug that your doctor is comfortable prescribing, and you have heard about it (from another patient, an advertisement, or online research) ask her about it. Not only will you save yourself quite a bit of money, you may actually be providing useful information to your doctor who may be able to prescribe the less costly alternative to other patients. Maybe, just maybe, when she's writing a script for the next patient, she may remember that you asked, "Is there a generic, a bio-equivalent medication that's less expensive you could recommend?"

Let me say right here and now, not all medications are created equal. They may have different inert ingredients that impact the metabolism, the activity, and the efficacy of the drug. There are times you have to pay the price for the more expensive drug because it simply works better. But, if you need a colonoscopy, for example, your doctor may prescribe a colon prep medication to get your colon squeaky clean so that he or she can clearly see how you look inside. One prep costs approximately $86. Another one $14. Our doctor had written a script for the $86 one. He was totally unaware of the cost until we told him. Hopefully, the next patient will benefit from the cost savings when the doctor prescribes the less expense prep.

Some pharmaceutical companies distribute coupons to doctors to help defray the cost of a drug. You may see them in the waiting room or the rest room. If you're not on a government funded insurance program—Medicare or Medicaid—you're eligible to use one of those coupons when you fill a prescription at the pharmacy. If you don't see any coupons, ask the nurse or medical assistant. They're likely to know if there is one there or he or she may be able to request one for you.

As for major drug costs, you'll want to do some research to find out if there are any support or charitable organizations that provide financial aid. If you Google your illness, those support organizations will show up. Contact these groups by phone or email to ask if they provide financial assistance. If they don't have financial assistance, ask if they can refer you to an organization that does offer aid. I've had to ask for financial assistance for oral cancer drugs which are incredibly expensive even with insurance coverage. Some of the charitable organizations will also provide some money for travel expenses or lodging.

Charitable organizations run out of money, if they don't get enough donor support. Fortunately, there are usually several organizations focusing on particular illnesses so you can contact another group, if necessary. It's also worth contacting an organization again after you've been turned down. Funds come and go. The organization may have run out of funding on Tuesday, but on Wednesday, a generous donor may show up and refill the coffers. It's certainly worth one more phone call or email to check on the status of the funds.

Another way to avoid some of the cost of drugs is to ask whether your doctor has any pharmaceutical samples in her office. Obviously, physicians won't have samples of every possible medication (chemotherapy drugs are not sampled), but if you can get an initial supply, that can be incredibly helpful. When I was a pharmaceutical representative, a physician would occasionally contact me to ask my company to provide free chemotherapy drugs for a patient. It was only for the most expensive medications and limited to those patients in dire circumstances. Sometimes, it's may be that a patient's insurance company simply won't pay for the drug or a procedure.

As a patient, it can be very frustrating finding financial aid when you're dealing with health issues. I understand. You might want to enlist the help of a friend or family member to help you sort through the maze of paperwork. There are people who are dedicated health-care advocates who charge for their services, but their assistance can lower your stress and frustration plus save you a great deal of time. A social worker in the hospital, a nurse or medical assistant in your doctor's office, are the best people to help you locate what you need. Don't give up too easily. It's worth the effort.

SMART ADVICE

◆ Ask your doctor if there's a less expensive drug that's bio-equivalent. Often doctors are truly unaware of the cost of drugs they prescribe.

◆ Coupons in your physicians' office can reduce the cost of some drugs. However, you are ineligible to use those coupons if you're on Medicare or Medicaid.

- Google your illness to find a support/charitable organization. These organizations often provide financial aid to patients with financial difficulties.

- If a support organization denies your request, check back in the future. The fund may be replenished by generous donors tomorrow.

- Pharmaceutical companies may supply free drugs to patients who are in rare and dire circumstances. Patients who are in unexpected financial difficulty, or when an insurance company has denied coverage for the drugs, may be eligible for support from the manufacturer (a pharmaceutical company).

- Nurses in the doctor's office or social workers in a hospital generally can guide you, if you need financial assistance. Explain your situation and ask for help. Why wait?

CHAPTER 18

Final Plans

Final plans—You know, the ones no one wants to talk about. The truth is we're all going and we're not going to the movies! Our passing may be many years from now or tomorrow, but the end of life is merely one more part of life itself.

A doctor who specializes in palliative care suggested I include a discussion about final plans in my book. She has dealt with many people who are at the end of their lives and haven't taken the time to put together a final plan. Not having a plan complicates our end of life journey and creates lots of unanswered questions for both physicians and family members when the time comes.

Exactly, what is a final plan? Here are the components that you may want to consider.

An Advance Medical Directive (which includes a Living Will and a Medical Power of Attorney). An Advanced Medical Directive is an end of life document that communicates your healthcare choices, if you're unable to. Most Advance Medical Directives include a section on organ donation where you can make your desires—to donate or not—very clear. That decision, that choice can be amended at any time.

Medical Power of Attorney—A designated person to make medical decisions for you should you be unable to do so.

End of Life Housing (Assisted Living, Care at Home—Long Term Care Insurance, etc.) Various living situations depending on the level of care you need. Long Term Care Insurance covers personal services and non-skilled nursing care at home and/or in other living circumstances.

Estate Plan (prepared by an attorney)—An advance plan compiled before you pass that includes beneficiaries of valuables, property, guardianship of young children, funeral wishes, tax and financial directives, etc.

A Will (You can do that by yourself or with the help of an attorney)—A legal document that instructs the care of your children and property when you die. It doesn't cover community property, life insurance payouts, tax liability, retirement assets and investment accounts.

Documents to Organize and Share (If you have investments, bonds, annuities, retirement accounts, bank and credit union accounts—any documents relating to those would be helpful.)

Additionally, personal property you'd like to pass on to someone special—furniture, vehicle, jewelry with the appropriate titles/appraisals, etc., if available.

Durable Power of Attorney—A legal document that allows a designated person to act on your behalf, if you're mentally incompetent, until you return to competency.

Funeral Plans—Type of burial, church/synagogue/mosque or any other venue of your choosing, a funeral home, cremation, casket, even music and flower selections can be noted.

Obituary and Death Notice—Would you like to write your own or have someone dear to you write it?

I realize it's a painful subject to even think about, but consider it both a generous and thoughtful endeavor for your survivors. In addition, it's the road map medical professionals will need to efficiently and professionally navigate your journey ahead. Oftentimes, patients are reluctant to bring it up in their doctor's office until it's absolutely necessary. But, even if you're one who truly thinks ahead and brings it up somewhat casually to your doctor, you may need to schedule an appointment solely dedicated to an end of life plan discussion. If your doctor doesn't ever bring up the topic, you should. Simply opening the door to that discussion will help you become more comfortable considering an end of life plan that works for you.

Obviously, there are no right or wrong plans. Each of our plans is individual and unique. If we haven't put together an end of life plan when it is just about the end of our life, that responsibility will fall on the shoulders of your kids, or your spouse/partner who will need to choose what they believe we'd want. And, even far more impersonal, if your family is unavailable or unable to decide what your final plans should be, a healthcare professional will be the one to do it. That's not ideal, certainly, but necessary.

Consider what you would like the end of your life to look like—each and every part of it. Talk with a family member or a dear friend. Speak with your doctor and an elder attorney if you can, but put together your plan—one that works for you.

SMART ADVICE:

- Talk with your physician about an end of life plan. It doesn't have to be complicated, but it should be a clear roadmap for your survivors and your physician to follow at the time of your passing.

- If you don't have one when your time is near, a plan will be put together by either your family (who will do what they "think" you would have wanted) or possibly by your physician who may not know your wishes.

- Your plan will be uniquely yours and spells out exactly your end of life choices. There are no right or wrong choices.

- If you physician doesn't bring up the discussion of end of life choices, you should bring it up. You may need to set up a visit specifically to discuss your needs in detail.

- Few of us want to think about or worse yet talk about dying. That said, an end of life plan removes some of the stress from an already, very difficult situation.

CHAPTER 19

You Know, You Look Really Good!

If I had a dollar for every time someone told me I looked really good during my cancer journey I might have enough money for a facelift! Only kidding—mostly! Seriously, when you're in treatment for any chronic disease or cancer, in particular, people don't know what to say. So, they try to say what they believe is supportive. Looking good = good health, right? Most people assume that if you look okay, you can't really be that sick. And, that's their hope—that you're going to be okay. It scares them to think otherwise.

There's this misperception that when people learn you have cancer or another serious illness they expect you to be in really dire shape or look absolutely awful. The good news is that for many people treatment for cancer or any other serious, chronic disease (that's why they call it chronic—it keeps on keepin' on—but is often manageable) can go on for years. Treatments can be quite stressful both physically and emotionally. But, currently, there are more treatments that are targeted (hitting the cancer/disease more directly with less damage to healthy, surrounding tissue) and tend not to be as debilitating.

That said, there are still some invasive treatments that are totally exhausting. I can relate. And these treatments can alter your appearance—hair loss (been there, done that with lots of turbans or nothing on my head at all), weight loss or weight gain, fatigue, etc. These changes in your appearance is what most people expect to see when they look at a chronically ill patient. For those patients, love and support as they go through such a difficult time is most helpful.

And, what about the rest of us who are handling treatments pretty well at the moment?

Don't be surprised if we actually do look really good! When I was a patient in a clinical trial at the National Cancer Institute I made it a point to wear a little makeup, keep my hair/clothes attractive, yet easy-care so I would feel less like a patient. There is definitely some truth to the old adage, "look good, feel good." As an oncology representative for a pharmaceutical company long before I was a patient myself we used to offer look good feel good seminars. Hiring a beauty consultant to do make-up and hairstyles for patients who were beautiful, just not feeling very beautiful at the time, really lifted their spirits. Even if only temporarily, a little emotional lift that takes people away from being a full-time patient offers a worthwhile change of pace. It's easy to forget who you were and what you looked like before the changes treatment often brings. Every reminder that your old self is still there and the hope that you'll be back to who you were is a necessary, positive, super-duper important and reinforcing belief.

Judging people's health based on their appearance is a reliable diagnostic tool used by doctors for centuries. It can sometimes tell more about a patient's health status than high tech equipment. In fact, the older doctors rely far more heavily on looking and listening to a patient than a CT scan, MRI, etc. My point is that if physicians choose appearance as a diagnostic tool, most people do too.

For me, I heard, "you know, you look really good," so often that I began to laugh every time someone said it, which was every day when I was in treatment or had a transplant. One friend, with a great sense of humor, used to say, "you know, you look like shit"—just to give me a laugh! To this day he would probably still say the same to see my reaction.

You may want to consider the fact that just because someone looks well doesn't always mean the person is feeling his or her best. Many are suffering, but their appearance belies their experience. I've had several, well meaning friend/family members tell me I was depressed while I was actually suffering the effects of early disease. I was also told I wasn't busy enough! But after I began listening to other patients and learned they had many days of fatigue, feeling down in the dumps, aches and pains during their early disease phase, I began to understand I wasn't actually depressed, but feeling lousy because I was ill.

Please don't assume that people are feeling well just because they look good. Not every ailment or treatment impacts appearance. Be kind, thoughtful, and offer any help you can.

SMART ADVICE

- Most people—healthcare providers, friends and family—will judge your health based on your appearance. Remember that not everyone who looks great is feeling the same.

CHAPTER 20

Positive Support for Patients (What You Can Do, What to Say or Not Say)

In addition to hearing "you know, you look really good," I've often heard these words, "Call me/let me know if there's anything I can do." I know people mean well, but it's pretty uncomfortable for most of us who have been patients to call our friends with a shopping list. Most of the time patients say, "I'm okay. I don't need anything." They do need help, but they're just too shy or proud to ask.

Fortunately, I have a wonderful husband who is willing to do just about anything (that's *just about anything*) to help. Therefore, I can simply ask for his help.

But, for other patients who don't have families or have a partner working three jobs just to pay for their healthcare insurance, they need some help. If you'd truly like to assist patients with day-to-day chores that they can't perform right now, be very specific. Offer to drive them to a doctor's appointment for a check-up or for a treatment. Ask if they'd like a ride both ways and would they like you to stay with them or not when they see the doctor or during treatment. A ride might be enough. Do they have a dog? Tell them when you'll be over to walk the dog today and for the next several days. Would they consider leaving the door open for you so you can pick up the dog without disturbing them? If it's grass-growing season, when is a good time of day to stop by and mow the lawn, as needed, in the next few months? How about an offer of babysitting even for an hour or so? That would be a great chance for someone who's not feeling their best to squeeze in a quick nap. Now that's a skill I've perfected since I've been in treatment, a nap, that is! You can always tell people you'll be over in an hour or so to pick up their grocery list. How about asking what they can eat? On a restricted diet? Best to ask before you begin cooking your world-famous chili for them! With that in mind, bringing the family a meal or two is always welcomed. Or, maybe they'd like to have a change of pace and go out for lunch or a movie. Offer to pick them up and allow them to spend a few hours not thinking about treatment.

By now, I'm sure you get my point. I can't stress enough the importance of volunteering for a specific chore with times and dates included. If you simply ask if and when you can do this or that for a person, he or she will very likely and very proudly turn you down. But, if you phrase your offer specifically and assertively, just about every person will accept your generous offer of help.

And, here's a huge thank you from all the current patients. Your help is very much appreciated.

And, one more thought: Please don't share the challenging experiences and deaths of other patients who've had the same illness that your friend/family member is undergoing now. Although, a patient may be doing well presently the fear of what can happen next is always in the back of their minds.

SMART ADVICE

* Forget the "call me, if there's anything I can do" offer. Most people who need some help won't call you either because of pride or a stubborn independence. Regardless, don't expect a phone call with a request for a specific chore you can do for them.

* Sincerely offered specific help will more than likely be accepted. Suggestions include driving people to the doctor or hospitals, babysitting, grocery shopping, dog walking or mowing the lawn.

* Ask the patient to consider leaving the door unlocked so you don't disturb him or her when you come by to help.

* Give him or her enough time—an hour or so or even the day before—to write up a shopping list before you plan to go to the market for them.

- Ask about diet restrictions before you cook up your famous duck a l'orange. He may not love it or just be unable to eat it.

- Stay in touch with offers to help whenever you can. I promise the patient will be very appreciative of whatever you can do.

Sources

"You want the person with the most experience in treating your specific condition, says Dr. Makary"— Page 80, *What Hospitals Won't Tell You and How Transparency Can Revolutionize Health Care, Marty Makary, MD,* Bloomsbury Press, 2012. Chapter 4.

"Promise me you'll always remember: You're braver than you believe, and stronger than you seem, and smarter than you think." Christopher Robin to Winnie The Poo.

Winnie The Pooh, A. A. Milne, Methuen & Company, Ltd., 1926.

Johns Hopkins Study—Deaths Due to Medical Errors, BMJ 2016; 353:i 2139, Dr. Marty Makary, Dr. Michael Daniel.

About the Author

Reina S. Weiner is a Healthcare and Patient Advocacy Coach, a former National Oncology Trainer and Nursing Instructor, multi-book author and presently a cancer patient in remission. Reina's previous book, *Strong From the Start—Raising Confident and Resilient Kids*—is available on Amazon.